Review Questions for I

Review Questions for MRI

Second Edition

Carolyn Kaut Roth, RT (R) (MR) (CT) (M) (CV) FSMRT

CEO, Imaging Education Associates, LLC
Berwyn, PA, USA

William H. Faulkner Jr, BS RT (R) (MR) (CT)

FSMRT

CEO, William Faulkner and Associates, LLC
Chattanooga, TN, USA

WILEY-BLACKWELL

A John Wiley & Sons, Ltd., Publication

Registered office: John Wiley & Sons, Ltd, The Atrium, Southern Gate, Chichester, West Sussex, PO19 8SQ, UK

Editorial offices: 9600 Garsington Road, Oxford, OX4 2DQ, UK
The Atrium, Southern Gate, Chichester, West Sussex, PO19 8SQ, UK
111 River Street, Hoboken, NJ 07030-5774, USA

For details of our global editorial offices, for customer services and for information about how to apply for permission to reuse the copyright material in this book please see our website at www.wiley.com/wiley-blackwell.

Library of Congress Cataloging-in-Publication Data
Roth, Carolyn Kaut.
  Review questions for MRI / Carolyn Kaut Roth, William H. Faulkner. – 2nd ed.
     p. ; cm.
  Includes bibliographical references and index.
  ISBN 978-1-4443-3390-9 (pbk. : alk. paper)
  I. Faulkner, William H. II. Title.
  [DNLM: 1. Magnetic Resonance Imaging–Examination Questions.   WN 18.2]
  616.07'548076–dc23
                          2012037037

A catalogue record for this book is available from the British Library.

Cover image: From left to right – Courtesy of tobkatrina; Selimakan; iStockphoto and HadelProductions
Cover design by Steve Thompson

Set in Times 10/12.5 pt Times by Toppan Best-set Premedia Limited
Printed and bound by CPI Group (UK) Ltd, Croydon, CR0 4YY

C9781444333909_140524

Contents

The contents specified within this publication are based upon:

- Content Specifications for the ARRT (American Registry of Radiologic Technologists) registry examination in MRI and as such remain ARRT's copyright
- Technologist Examination Overview for the ARMRIT (American Registry for MRI Technologists) registry examination in MRI and as such remain ARMRIT's copyright
- Radiographer Advanced Examination in MRI for the CAMRT (Canadian Medical Radiographer Technologist) registry examination in MRI and as such remain CAMRT's copyright

Preface

Beginning with the acquisition of the first clinical MR image and continuing into the present, the principles of magnetic resonance technology have continued to confound even the academics. In response to complex imaging principles, many MR system users, mostly technologists, had given up any hope of ever learning the fundamentals of MRI. For this reason, the level of expertise of MRI technologists varies greatly between imaging centers. In response to the remarkable difference in proficiency and level of understanding, a need emerged for the standardization of MRI practitioner skills. That need was met by several accrediting agencies with the implementation of advanced-level examinations in MRI, known as the "MRI Boards". Also, in an attempt to maintain "high-quality diagnostic imaging centers" in MRI, The American College of Radiology (ACR) has implemented "site accreditation" for MRI facilities. These ACR standards include "site standards" for the facility as well as "minimum requirements" for MRI technologists. Recommendations include technologist/radiographer certification. To date, the ACR recognizes several accrediting agencies (advanced-level examinations in MRI) for technologists, including those exams offered by:

- The American Registry for Radiologic Technologists (ARRT)
- The ARMRIT (American Registry for MRI Technologists)
- The CAMRT (Canadian Medical Radiographer Technologist)

With the introduction of advanced-level examinations for MRI, technologists actively involved in MRI are looking for resource materials that will prepare them for these examinations. After facing numerous requests for registry review materials, we decided to combine and expand on the examination questions and answers that we have used effectively for the past 20+ years in each of our teaching programs. The result of this compilation was presented here as *Review Questions for MRI*, first edition. As MRI continues to evolve, we take the liberty to "update" the material within this study guide to provide the technologist or radiographer with up-to-date study materials. This second edition will provide the user with a comprehensive review of the principles and applications of MRI to prepare practicing MRI technologists for the advanced-level examination.

This book is intended for those technologists who are actively involved in MRI and/ or those who have completed a training program in MRI and intend to sit for an advanced-level registry examination. This Q & A book is filled with multiple choice and True/False questions and answers that follow the topics listed in the content specifications offered by the ARRT, the examination overview by the ARMRIT, and the CAMRT guidelines.

Who will benefit from this book?

This book will serve the needs for any technologist who is preparing for the boards, including:

- The technologist who is working in MRI and who has never had the opportunity to attend formal didactic (classroom) training, but whose employment requires that they must take and pass the Boards.
- The technologist who has recently completed a formal training program in MRI and is preparing for the Boards.

For those technologists who are preparing for their examinations, this resource will be helpful for:

- The technologist who has completed their studies and wants to "reinforce" what they have already studied, prior to taking the examination. . . .
  "The icing on the cake" so to speak!
- The technologist who has begun their studies and would like to "identify" their strengths and weaknesses in MRI theory during the study process and prior to taking the examination . . .
  "The cake"
- The technologist who has not yet begun their studies, but who is overwhelmed by the principles of MRI and would like to know "where to begin" . . .
  "The recipe for the cake"

For the record, we (Bill and Candi) are not on any of the ARRT, CAMRT, or ARMRIT committees for the registry examinations, nor are we privy to any inside information regarding the examination. Therefore, these questions are ones that have been used for previous educational programs, classroom tests, quizzes, and final examinations, as well as questions written explicitly for this publication. Any similarities between this book and the registry examination are, therefore, purely coincidental. However, having taught MRI principles and applications for the past several years, and since the content specifications themselves closely resemble our program outlines, the material covered within this review book should serve as an adequate study guide for the advanced-level examinations in MRI, also known as the MRI Boards.

Acknowledgements

First, I must thank God for the knowledge to complete this educational offering. Second, and always, I need to thank my family, friends, and my loving husband, Scott, for their support. Next, I would like to include within my "thank you list" all of hard working personnel, colleagues, and friends from Imaging Education Associates (IEA) including: my associates PJ, Pat R, Amy; my faculty and professional colleagues Joy, Wil, Barb, and the IEA faculty. Finally, I must thank all of the technologists, radiologists, nurses, and corporate personnel that I have had the opportunity to "teach". In fact, teaching these healthcare professionals has had a boomerang effect whereby they have actually "taught" me! It also goes without saying that it has been my privilege to have worked with Bill Faulkner on this and many other projects for over 25 years. I am honored to have been a part of your professional lives. May God bless you as you study for your boards!

Candi

I suppose that with a name like William Faulkner, it was inevitable that it should wind up on the front of a book. That said, since I am William Faulkner, Jr, I want to thank my parents not only for the name, but also for the support, encouragement, and love I still receive. I also want to thank and acknowledge my wife, Tricia, our daughter, Amber, her husband Ricky, and now our beautiful and wonderful granddaughter Zooey Ann for their love and support. (You can only imagine what I'm like to live with.) It would be remiss if I did not thank the unequaled group of radiologists and technologists with whom I have the pleasure of working with over the years. (You can only imagine what I'm like to work with.) In particular, I want to thank the late Dr James Crawley, who offered me my first job in MRI, and Dr Don Mills who then had to work with me while I began learning MRI. Dr Mills gave his time and energy to offer me an education that could not be given a price; I am eternally grateful. I have truly been blessed to meet and work with many wonderful professionals over the course of my career. It should be obvious that my participation in this book would not have been possible without having the great fortune to meet and work with Candi Roth. Every job has its ups and downs and we are not always happy. However, because of these great people and many others, I can say that l have always enjoyed my career. Finally, I want to thank God, for without Him, nothing would be possible.

Bill

Introduction

Magnetic resonance imaging (MRI) is a diagnostic imaging modality that is used to evaluate anatomic structures and pathologic conditions within the body. MRI is known for its exquisite demonstration of soft tissues within the body. For this reason, the majority of MR imaging is performed for the evaluation of hydrogen. Hydrogen atoms behave like a microscopic magnet when exposed to the strong magnetic field associated with MR imaging. For this reason, hydrogen is said to be "MR active". In addition, the human body is approximately 75% water. The combination of the *relative* abundance of hydrogen within the body and the magnetic characteristics of the hydrogen atom explains the utilization of hydrogen for MR imaging. Although other substances can be evaluated with magnetic resonance, hydrogen is typically preferred. It is the hydrogen in water (H_2O or two hydrogens bound to one oxygen) and the hydrogen in fat (CH_3 or three hydrogens bound to one carbon) that represent the substances typically evaluated by magnetic resonance. This evaluation can be provided by imaging (known as magnetic resonance imaging – MRI) and/or magnetic resonance spectroscopy (MRS). MRI and/or MRS can be performed on a specimen *in vivo* (within the body) or *in vitro* (outside the body, e.g. within a test tube).

To acquire MR or MRS images, a complex combination of hardware and software components are required. As the name implies, the MR imager consists of several different types of magnets. Magnets used in MRI include permanent magnets and electromagnets. Electromagnets include resistive and superconducting magnets. Resistive magnets can be used to create the main magnetic field and/or other magnetic system components. Permanent, resistive, and superconducting magnets can create various types of magnetic fields: "static" magnetic fields and "time-varying" magnetic fields. Magnets that produce static magnetic fields create magnetic fields that are "unchanging". The static magnetic field associated with the main magnet is known as the B_0 field. Magnets that produce time-varying magnetic fields (TVMF) create magnetic fields that that "vary" or "change" over time. TVMF are associated with RF fields and/or gradient fields. Oscillating magnetic fields, such as the radiofrequency (RF) field, are employed during imaging acquisition, known as excitation. This secondary (oscillating) magnetic field is known as the B_1 field. TVMF are also associated with magnetic fields that are switched on and off over time. Gradient magnetic fields produce a linear "gradation" or slope in the magnetic field that is switched on and off during image acquisition. The primary function of gradient magnetic fields is spatial encoding, allowing for various imaging planes (or views) to be acquired without moving the patient.

Various magnetic components such as RF and gradients are "pulsed" on and off during MR image acquisition. The sequence of these "pulses" determines the type of image that is acquired during MR imaging. This is known as a "pulse sequence". Computers are programmed to "direct" the various magnets within the MR imager to coordinate their usage during MR image acquisition. MR images can be acquired with various types of imaging planes (views) and/or with different types of image contrast (known as T1-, T2-, or proton density-weighted images). For example, images can be acquired whereby the fat is bright and water dark (T1-weighted image), or by changing imaging parameters (technique factors), images can be acquired whereby the water is bright and fat darker (T2-weighted image). Each patient is evaluated with several different types of images (various imaging planes or views), and/or acquisitions with different image contrast (different image weighting). The combination of images acquired for a patient is known as a protocol. The protocol consists of images acquired with various views or planes (sagittal, axial, coronal, and/or oblique) with various contrast or weighting (T1-, T2-, proton density-weighting), depending upon the anatomy and pathology to be imaged.

Each type of magnet within the MR imager functions differently. For this reason, each MR system component has unique safety considerations. To date there are no known, long-term biologic effects associated with exposure to the magnetic field. The safety consideration associated with the static magnetic field (specifically the stray field or fringe field located outside the MR imager) is generally associated with forces (translational force and rotational force) resulting in "projectiles" and "torque". Even though MR imaging does not use "ionizing" radiation, imaging does require radiofrequency (RF) energy that is considered to be low energy or "nonionizing" radiation. The Food and Drug Administration (FDA) imposes limits on exposure to various components of the MR imager, including the static field, RF field, and gradient magnetic field. Because of these various and unique magnetic field effects, patient care and safety in the MR environment is critical.

The technologist who operates the MR imager should understand all of the aspects of MR imaging. These aspects include: the MR system components (hardware or instrumentation); safety associated with these system components; the substances that can be imaged by MR (hydrogen and other elements); the method by which MR images are acquired (imaging planes and image weighting); and the anatomy (and pathology) to be imaged. In order to evaluate the knowledge of the MRI technologist, the American Registry for Radiologic technologists (ARRT) has developed an advanced-level examination in MRI. This has been divided into four categories:

- Patient care in MRI (general patient care and MRI safety)
- Imaging procedures (cross-sectional anatomy and clinical applications for MRI and contrast-enhanced MR)
- Data acquisition and processing (pulse sequences, parameters, and options for MR image formation)
- Physical principles of image formation (MR instrumentation and fundamentals for image acquisition).

To provide the technologist with information about the advanced-level examination in MRI, the ARRT has provided a document known as the "content specifications" (or content specs). This outlines the topics and subtopics that will be tested in the examination. Essentially, the content specifications "hint" as to the categories of questions (topics), the information for the questions (subtopics), and the number of questions (per category) that will be included in the advanced-level examination for MRI. The table of contents (and the outline below it) reflects the "topics and subtopics" associated with the content specs. These documents are updated periodically; therefore, it is always recommended to visit the ARRT website for the most current version of the content specifications (www.arrt.org).

This book is designed to provide the technologist with questions associated with the content specifications provided by the ARRT. This book contains four parts that match the four main "topics" associated with the content specs. Within each part are subtopics to help technologist prepare for the MRI Boards.

Part A

Patient Care in MRI

Bioeffects, Safety, and Patient Care

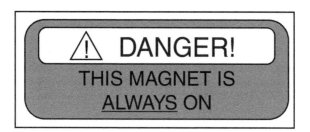

Introduction

To date, there are no known long-term biological effects associated with magnetic resonance imaging (MRI). However, there are some aspects of MRI that could potentially
result in irreversible and devastating outcomes for the patients and operators. These
aspects include the static magnetic fields (potential projectiles and torque), the time-
varying magnetic fields associated with the magnetic field gradients (peripheral nerve
stimulation and acoustic noise), and the radiofrequency field (thermal injuries, heating,
and burns). Part A will provide "practice" questions to prepare for the safety component
of the MRI Boards.

MR image acquisition is very different from radiographic imaging, nuclear medicine,
and sonography. The instrumentation used and the physical principles of image formation
are "unique" for MR imaging. For these reasons, safety considerations for patients and
personnel in MRI are also "unique" to the modality. For example, the strength of the
magnetic field in the majority of MR imagers is so high (1.5 Tesla or 10000 Gauss) that
terminal velocity of a "paperclip" is up to 40 miles per hour. A simple paperclip would
hit the side of the MR scanner at 40 mph! Furthermore, the velocity with which a metallic
object (such as the paperclip) flies toward the scanner is determined by the mass of the
object and the distance from the scanner (in addition to the type of metal and strength
of the magnetic field). One can only imagine the damage that could be done if an oxygen

Review Questions for MRI, Second Edition. Carolyn Kaut Roth and William H. Faulkner.
© 2013 Carolyn Kaut Roth and William S. Faulkner. Published 2013 by Blackwell Publishing Ltd.

tank was inadvertently brought into the MR scan room. MR safety can be a "life-or-death" scenario. Part A will provide practice questions about projectiles (flying metallic objects) as well as other "life-threatening" safety considerations in MRI.

The safety component of the MRI Boards (post primary examination and/or primary examination)

Beginning in 1995, the advanced-level examination in MRI was available as a "post primary examination". At that time, the post primary examination was only available for the registered technologist in radiography (RT (R)). To qualify for the MRI (post primary) examination, the technologist had to have a "primary certification". The primary examination could include: the radiography examination (RT (R)), the nuclear medicine examination (RT(N)), and the radiation therapy examination (RT (T)) or the sonography examination RT (S)). The assumption was that the technologist had already learned (and had been tested on) subjects such as "general patient care" during their primary examination. Therefore, when the MRI Boards were only available as a post primary examination, the safety category of the MRI boards included *only* MRI safety considerations.

Toward the fall of 2005 the ARRT announced that "the technologist need not be an *RT* to qualify for the advanced level examination in MRI". In January 2006, the ARRT defined the statement whereby one could qualify for the exam as a primary examination or a post primary examination. To qualify for the post primary examination, the technologist must have a primary certification (explained above). To qualify for the "primary examination", the "student" must attend an accredited MRI educational program. This program "can" resemble a radiography program, whereby the radiation physics is replaced by MR physics; radiation technique is replaced by MRI scan parameters; and patient care and radiation safety is replaced by patient care and MR safety. Today the MRI Boards are available as a "post primary examination" (for the RT) and also as a "primary examination" (for the non-RT). For this reason, the safety category within the advanced-level examination in MRI includes not only MRI safety but also general patient care.

There are several types of examination for the MRI technologist in North America, including the ARRT examination, the ARMRIT examination, and the CAMRT examination. Each examination has safety questions and these make up roughly 15–20% of the examination.

Part A offers review questions and answers that relate to general patient care and MRI safety considerations. Even though the questions are set with the guidelines from the content specifications from North American Boards in mind, MRI safety is critical for healthcare workers in the MR environment worldwide!

General patient care

1. Legal and ethical principles
   a. Confirmation of exam requisition
   b. Legal issues

    c. Patient's rights

    d. ARRT standard of ethics

2. Patient assessment, monitoring, and management

    a. Routine monitoring

    b. Emergency response

    c. Patient transfer and body mechanics

    d. Assisting patients with medical equipment

3. Interpersonal communications

    a. Modes of communication

    b. Challenges in communication

    c. Patient education

    d. Medical terminology

4. Infection control

    a. Terminology and basic concepts

    b. Cycle of infection

    c. Standard precautions (general patient contact)

    d. Additional or transmission-based precautions (e.g. hepatitis B, HIV, tuberculosis)

    e. Disposal of contaminated materials

Legal and ethical principles

It is important for the MRI technologist to understand legal and ethical issues associated with MR imaging. This information is critical as deviation from these standards can lead to unsafe patient practices, lawsuits, and/or termination of employment. Questions on legal and ethical principles are drawn from the following subject areas:

a. Confirmation of exam requisition

    i. Verification of patient identification

    ii. Comparison of request to clinical indications

b. Legal issues

    i. Common terminology (e.g. negligence, malpractice)

    ii. Legal doctrines (e.g. *respondeat superior, res ipsa loquitur*)

c. Patient's rights

    i. Informed consent (written, oral, implied)

    ii. Confidentiality (HIPAA)

    iii. Patient's Bill of Rights (e.g. privacy, access to information, healthcare proxy, research participation)

d. Standard of ethics

    i. ARRT

    ii. CAMRT

    iii. ARMRIT

Questions 1–29 concern legal and ethical principles.

Patient assessment, monitoring, and management

This category has been modified from the original content specifications and includes patient management information. Questions on patient assessment, monitoring, and assessment are drawn from the following subject areas:

a. Routine monitoring
   i. Vital signs
   ii. Physical signs and symptoms
   iii. Sedated patients
   iv. Claustrophobic patients

b. Emergency response
   i. Reactions to contrast
   ii. Other allergic reactions (e.g. latex)
   iii. Cardiac/respiratory arrest (CPR)
   iv. Physical injury, trauma, or RF burn
   v. Other medical disorders (e.g. seizures, diabetic reactions)
   vi. Life-threatening situations (e.g. quench, projectiles)

c. Patient transfer and body mechanics

d. Assisting patients with medical equipment
   i. Implantable devices (e.g. infusion catheters, pumps, pacemakers, others)
   ii. Oxygen delivery systems
   iii. Other (e.g. nasogastric tubes, urinary catheters)

Questions 30–104 concern patient assessment, monitoring, and management.

Interpersonal communications

Since the advanced-level examination offered by the ARRT is now available as a primary examination (for the person who attended an accredited MRI school) or a post primary examination [for the technologist who first studied a primary modality such as radiography RT (R), or nuclear medicine RT (N), or radiation therapy RT (T)], new patient care information has been added to the content specifications. Questions on communication are drawn from the following subject areas:

a. Modes of communication
   i. Verbal, written
   ii. Nonverbal (e.g. eye contact, touching)

b. Challenges in communication
   i. Patient characteristics (e.g. cultural factors, physical or emotional status)
   ii. Strategies to improve understanding

c. Patient education
   i. Explanation of procedure (e.g. risks, benefits)
   ii. Follow-up instructions
   iii. Referral to other services

d. Medical terminology

Questions 105–114 concern interpersonal communications.

Infection control

Since the advanced-level examination offered by the ARRT is now available as a primary examination (for the person who attended an accredited MRI school) or a post primary examination [for the technologist who first studied a primary modality such as radiography RT (R), or nuclear medicine RT (N), or radiation therapy RT (T)], new patient care information has been added to the content specifications. Questions on infection control are drawn from the following subject areas:

a. Terminology and basic concepts
  i. Types of asepsis
  ii. Sterile technique
  iii. Pathogens (e.g. fomites, vehicles, vectors)
  iv. Nosocomial infections

b. Cycle of infection
  i. Pathogen
  ii. Source or reservoir of infection
  iii. Susceptible host
  iv. Method of transmission (contact, droplet, airborne, common vehicle, vector borne)

c. Standard precautions (general patient contact)
  i. Handwashing
  ii. Gloves, gowns
  iii. Masks
  iv. Medical asepsis/disinfection

d. Additional or transmission-based precautions (e.g. hepatitis B, HIV, tuberculosis)
  i. Airborne (e.g. negative ventilation)
  ii. Droplet (e.g. particulate mask)
  iii. Contact (e.g. gloves, gown)

e. Disposal of contaminated materials
  i. Linens
  ii. Needles
  iii. Patient supplies
  Questions 115–138 concern infection control.

MRI screening and safety

This category is from the original (ARRT post primary) examination. Questions on MRI screening and safety are drawn from the following subject areas. (The ARMRIT and the CAMRT also have MRI screening and safety categories within their examinations.)

1. Biological effects and MRI safety considerations
   a. RF field
      i. Specific absorption rate (SAR)
      ii. Biological effects
      iii. FDA guidelines
   b. Static and gradient magnetic fields
      i. Biological effects
      ii. FDA guidelines
   c. Acoustic noise

2. MRI screening, monitoring, and assessment
   a. Screening
      i. Biomedical implants (e.g. pacemakers, clips)
      ii. Ferrous foreign bodies
      iii. Medical conditions
      iv. Prior diagnostic or surgical procedures
   b. Equipment safety
      i. Placement of conductors (e.g. ECG leads, coils, cables)
      ii. Cryogen safety
      iii. Ancillary equipment in proximity
      iv. Emergency procedures (e.g. quench, fire)
   c. Environment
      i. Climate control (temperature, humidity)
      ii. Gauss lines
      iii. Magnetic shielding
      iv. RF shielding
      v. American Registry for Radiologic technologists Warning signs

Questions 139–202 concern MRI screening and safety.

Part A: Questions

Legal and ethical principles

1. What is the first duty the technologist should perform when beginning an MR examination?

   a. Check the physician's orders in the chart ☐
   b. Verify the patient's identity ☐
   c. Place the film in the Bucky tray ☐
   d. Obtain an accurate medical history on the patient ☐

2. In a medical malpractice suit, the _____ must prove medical malpractice.

   a. Physician charged ☐
   b. Risk manager ☐
   c. Patient plaintiff ☐
   d. Technologist performing the scan ☐

3. Healthcare workers generally practice _____, which states the "goal is to do no harm".

   a. Beneficence ☐
   b. Confidentiality ☐
   c. Nonmaleficence ☐
   d. The prudent professional standard ☐

4. A patient on the MRI table is left unattended and rolls off onto the floor, causing an injury to the head. The technologist in attendance can be sued for:

   a. Slander ☐
   b. Negligence ☐
   c. Battery ☐
   d. False imprisonment ☐

5. A patient, deemed competent, becomes claustrophobic during an MRI procedure and refuses to continue with the study. The technologist should first:

   a. Call for security and force the patient to continue ☐
   b. Stop the study and inform the supervisor ☐
   c. Coerce the patient to be more cooperative ☐
   d. Reassure the patient and attempt to talk him or her through the procedure ☐

6. A malpractice case based on an obvious negligent act, e.g. a radiograph (or MR image) of the abdomen demonstrates that a surgical sponge was inadvertently left in the surgical site (within the peritoneum) after surgery, will likely be considered under the doctrine of:

a. *Respondeat superior*	☐
b. *Res ipsa loquitor*	☐
c. *Stare decisis*	☐
d. Breach of confidentiality	☐

7. When entering data on a patient's chart, the technologist must be sure to:

a. Sign and date the entry	☐
b. Date the entry, record the time, and sign using name and credentials	☐
c. Date the entry, record the time, and indicate your department	☐
d. Date the entry and sign using name and credentials	☐

8. Unintentional misconduct is also known as:

a. Libel	☐
b. Battery	☐
c. False imprisonment	☐
d. Negligence	☐

9. Which of the following describes assault of the patient?

a. Hitting the patient	☐
b. Restraining the patient	☐
c. Causing the patient to feel threatened	☐
d. Performing an MRI study against the patient's will	☐

10. Which of the following statements is incorrect regarding the principle of the double effect?

a. The action must be morally neutral or good	☐
b. The good effect is not the only intention	☐
c. The good effect must be equal to or greater in importance than the bad effect	☐
d. The bad effect must not be the means by which the good effect is accomplished	☐

11. An ambulatory, outpatient lying down on the MRI table as requested by the technologist has given:

> **a.** Implied consent ☐
> **b.** Informed consent ☐
> **c.** Emergency consent ☐
> **d.** Vicarious liability ☐

12. Which of the following is an example of battery?

> **a.** Threatening the patient ☐
> **b.** Sharing patient information with another technologist in the work area ☐
> **c.** Imaging the incorrect body part ☐
> **d.** Using an immobilization device ☐

13. Which is the most likely type of law under which a suit is brought against a technologist for performing unintentional acts that fall below the standard of care and result in patient injury?

> **a.** Felonious ☐
> **b.** Tort ☐
> **c.** Criminal ☐
> **d.** Administrative ☐

14. *Respondeat superior* is a Latin term meaning:

> **a.** The thing speaks for itself ☐
> **b.** The reasonable technologist should make the decision ☐
> **c.** There is no need for the MRI technologist to carry their own liability insurance ☐
> **d.** Let the master answer ☐

15. Which of the following is NOT a true statement regarding informed consent?

> **a.** Consent must be given under no duress ☐
> **b.** The patient must understand all aspects of the procedure being performed ☐
> **c.** The patient must be of legal age ☐
> **d.** The procedure must be explained in terms that the patient can understand, to include risks and benefits ☐

16. Destroying or altering medical records without legitimate authorization or reason is called:

a. Medical negligence ☐
b. Failure to follow standard of care ☐
c. Spoliation ☐
d. Vicarious liability ☐

17. Which of the following means "to stand by things decided"?

a. Consequentialism ☐
b. *Res ipsa loquitor* ☐
c. *Respondeat superior* ☐
d. *Stare decisis* ☐

18. A technologist who touches a patient without permission (with the exception of emergency consent) could be found guilty of:

a. Negligence ☐
b. Breach of confidentiality ☐
c. Battery ☐
d. Assault ☐

19. Discussing a patient's confidential medical information with a person who does not have a need to know is called:

a. Vicarious liability ☐
b. Invasion of privacy ☐
c. Libel ☐
d. *Stare decisis* ☐

20. If the supervising radiologist instructs you to scan a patient with a known cardiac pacemaker and the patient goes into cardiac arrest due to pacemaker failure, you MAY be protected from a lawsuit under the doctrine of *respondeat superior*, which means:

a. Let the master answer ☐
b. The thing speaks for itself ☐
c. Radiologists (like all supervising physicians) are always liable ☐
d. Hospital administration decides who is liable in each situation ☐

21. Patient rights would include all of the following EXCEPT:

> **a.** Right to privacy ☐
> **b.** Right to a diagnosis by the MRI technologist ☐
> **c.** Right to refuse the MRI study ☐
> **d.** Right to know potential risks of the MRI study ☐

22. Which of the following is the term used to describe written malicious spreading of information?

> **a.** Breach of confidentiality ☐
> **b.** Libel ☐
> **c.** Slander ☐
> **d.** Qualified privilege ☐

23. The burden of proof for medical negligence rests with the:

> **a.** Physician ☐
> **b.** Patient ☐
> **c.** Radiographer ☐
> **d.** Risk manager ☐

24. All of the following may be considered an example of battery EXCEPT:

> **a.** Touching the patient without consent ☐
> **b.** Sharing patient information with another technologist in the work area ☐
> **c.** Imaging the wrong body part ☐
> **d.** Restraining the patient ☐

25. Which of the following describes assault of the patient?

> **a.** Striking the patient ☐
> **b.** Touching the patient without consent ☐
> **c.** Threatening the patient or causing the patient to feel threatened ☐
> **d.** Performing a radiographic procedure against the patient's will ☐

26. The concept of the reasonable prudent person is interpreted as:

> **a.** How a reasonable jury member would perform the act ☐
> **b.** How a professional with similar education, training, and experience would perform the act ☐
> **c.** How a prudent attorney would interpret the act ☐
> **d.** How a reasonable and prudent judge will rule on the act ☐

27. According to the ARRT standard of ethics, the radiologic technologist acts to advance the principal objective of the profession to provide services to humanity _____.

- **a.** With full respect for the dignity of mankind ☐
- **b.** With discrimination on the basis of sex, race, creed, religion, or socio-economic status ☐
- **c.** Understanding interpretation and diagnosis are within the scope of practice for the profession ☐
- **d.** Providing full disclosure for all patient information among colleagues and other patients ☐

28. According to the ARRT standard of ethics (specifically within the Code of Ethics), the radiologic technologist acts to advance the principal objective of the profession to provide services to humanity and includes all of the following EXCEPT:

- **a.** The radiologic technologist conducts herself or himself in a professional manner, responds to patient needs, and supports colleagues and associates in providing quality patient care ☐
- **b.** The radiologic technologist acts to advance the principal objective of the profession to provide services to humanity with full respect for the dignity of mankind ☐
- **c.** Delivers patient care and service unrestricted by the concerns of personal attributes or the nature of the disease or illness, and without discrimination on the basis of sex, race, creed, religion, or socio-economic status ☐
- **d.** Practices technology founded upon theoretical knowledge and concepts, uses equipment and accessories inconsistent with the purposes for which they were designed, and employs procedures and techniques inappropriately ☐

29. Which of the following circumstances would NOT be an ARRT ethical violation?

- **a.** Contacting a referring doctor when he or she has ordered the wrong procedure on a patient ☐
- **b.** Discussing with your colleagues whether or not you should do the procedure if the order is incorrect ☐
- **c.** Performing the procedure on the patient if the order is not correct ☐
- **d.** Performing a procedure on a patient without any order ☐

Patient assessment, monitoring, and management

30. Which of the following may cause a patient to experience a syncopal episode?
  1. Anxiety
  2. Hunger
  3. Hypertension

a. 1 only	☐
b. 3 only	☐
c. 1 and 2 only	☐
d. 2 and 3 only	☐

31. All claustrophobic patients who are scheduled for MRI examinations should be:

a. Sedated	☐
b. Forced to overcome their fear to complete the examination	☐
c. Rescheduled for another day	☐
d. Handled delicately so as not to compound their anxiety	☐

32. Patients who should be monitored (with pulse oximetry) during MRI procedures are:
  1. Unresponsive and uncommunicative patients
  2. Sedated, psychiatric and pediatric patients
  3. Patients who have weak voices and/or impaired hearing

a. 1 only	☐
b. 1 and 2 only	☐
c. 1 and 3 only	☐
d. 1, 2, and 3	☐

33. Patients who have been sedated with diazepam should be monitored with:

a. Pulse oximetry	☐
b. ECG gating	☐
c. Peripheral gating	☐
d. Verbal communication	☐

34. It is good practice for all patients who undergo MRI to be monitored:

a. Visually and/or verbally	☐
b. By ECG	☐
c. By respiratory monitors	☐
d. Not at all	☐

35. BEFORE the publication of the "Contrast Media Update" by the ACR in 2010, contraindications for using gadolinium included:
1. Sickle cell crisis and hypertension
2. Pregnancy and breast-feeding mothers
3. High BUN and creatinine
4. Low GFR
5. Renal insufficiency and/or acute renal injury
6. None known

a. 6 only ☐
b. 1, 2, and 3 only ☐
c. 4 and 5 only ☐
d. 1, 2, 3, 4, and 5 only ☐

36. AFTER the publication of the first edition of the "Contrast Media Update" by the ACR in 2010, contraindications for using gadolinium included:
1. Sickle cell crisis and hypertension
2. Pregnancy and breast-feeding mothers
3. High BUN and creatinine
4. Low GFR
5. Renal insufficiency and/or acute renal injury
6. None known

a. 6 only ☐
b. 1, 2, and 3 only ☐
c. 4 and 5 only ☐
d. 1, 2, 3, 4, and 5 only ☐

37. Precautions for the use of gadolinium include:
1. Sickle cell crisis and hypertension
2. Pregnancy
3. Low GFR
4. Hemolytic anomalies and lactating mothers
5. Prior contrast reactions and patients with a history of asthma or allergies

a. 3 only ☐
b. 1, 2, and 3 only ☐
c. 2, 3, 4, and 5 only ☐
d. 1, 2, 3, 4, and 5 ☐

38. The approved gadolinium contrast agents are currently indicated for:
1. Intravenous injection for pediatric imaging
2. Intravenous injection for abdominal imaging
3. Intravenous injection for central nervous system (CNS) imaging
4. Intra-articular injection for musculoskeletal imaging

a. 3 only ☐
b. 2 and 3 only ☐
c. 1, 2, and 3 only ☐
d. 1, 2, 3, and 4 ☐

39. The patient who has too much insulin in their body is experiencing:

a. Diabetic coma ☐
b. Hyperglycemia ☐
c. Hypoglycemia ☐
d. Hypovolemia ☐

40. What is the correct order for administering basic life support?

a. Airway, breathing, circulation ☐
b. Circulation, breathing, airway ☐
c. Breathing, circulation, airway ☐
d. Airway, circulation, breathing ☐

41. If a patient, while recumbent on the MR couch, says that he or she feels "faint", what action should the technologist take?

a. Sit the patient upright slowly ☐
b. Contact the referring physician ☐
c. Place the patient in the Fowler's position ☐
d. Place the patient in the Trendelenberg position ☐

42. The proper method of treating contrast media extravasation is to:

a. Place a warm compress over the site and complete the contrast administration ☐
b. Remove the needle, place a bandage over the injection site to stop bleeding, and choose another location to complete the contrast administration ☐
c. Remove the needle, hold pressure on the vein until bleeding stops, then apply ice ☐
d. Stop the injection and wait for the fluid collection to disperse, then resume contrast administration ☐

43. Which of the following may cause a loss of patency in an IV line?

a. Using the incorrect IV solution ☐
b. Improper height of the IV solution ☐
c. Poor circulation ☐
d. Improper needle selection ☐

44. Deep veins are not used in venipuncture because:

    a. They are too difficult to locate ☐
    b. Their tunica intima is much thicker ☐
    c. They are close to major arteries and nerves ☐
    d. There would be possible interference with the lymphatic system ☐

45. Which of the following can be used for multiple doses of the same drug?

    a. Ampule ☐
    b. Vial ☐

46. Reducing viscosity of contrast media can be accomplished by:

    a. Warming the contrast prior to administration ☐
    b. Cooling the contrast prior to administration ☐
    c. Shaking the container vigorously prior to administration ☐
    d. Storing the container in an area with low humidity ☐

47. The stated gauge of the IV needle or catheter refers to its:

    a. Length ☐
    b. Bevel angle ☐
    c. Diameter ☐
    d. Circumference ☐

48. Which blood test for renal function is used in the calculation of eGFR (estimated glomerular filtration rate)?

    a. Blood urea nitrogen (BUN) ☐
    b. Hematocrit ☐
    c. Partial thromboplastin time ☐
    d. Serum creatinine ☐

49. Which of the following blood tests would NOT be used to assess the patient's risk of hemorrhaging during an invasive procedure (such as a biopsy)?

    a. Prothrombin time (PT) ☐
    b. Hematocrit ☐
    c. International normalized ratio (INR) ☐
    d. Platelet count ☐

50. Which blood vessel has the thickest tunica media?

> **a.** Artery ☐
> **b.** Vein ☐
> **c.** Capillary ☐
> **d.** Lymphatic ☐

51. A normal serum creatinine range is:

> **a.** 0.2–1.0 mg/dL ☐
> **b.** 0.6–1.5 mg/dL ☐
> **c.** 0.8–2.5 mg/dL ☐
> **d.** 1.2–3.0 mg/dL ☐

52. An eGFR of below 15 is indicative of:

> **a.** Normal kidney function ☐
> **b.** A kidney infection ☐
> **c.** Polycystic kidney ☐
> **d.** A patient in need of dialysis ☐

53. Although ALL patients must be evaluated on a case by case basis, the ACR recommends that gadolinium should not be administered in patients with an eGFR of:

> **a.** 50 and above ☐
> **b.** 30 and above ☐
> **c.** 30 and below ☐
> **d.** There is no relationship between eGFR and the administration of ☐
>   gadolinium contrast media

54. Which type of circulation is responsible for reoxygenation of the blood?

> **a.** Pulmonary ☐
> **b.** Systemic ☐
> **c.** Nonsystemic ☐
> **d.** Portal ☐

55. Which of the layers of a blood vessel is made of fibrous, connective tissue?

> **a.** Tunica adventitia ☐
> **b.** Tunica media ☐
> **c.** Tunica intima ☐
> **d.** Capillaries ☐

56. A normal range for blood urea nitrogen (BUN) is:

a. 0.6–1.5 mg/100 dL ☐
b. 2.0–15.0 mg/100 dL ☐
c. 8.0–20.0 mg/100 dL ☐
d. 25.0–50.0 mg/100 dL ☐

57. Which type of blood cell carries oxygenated hemoglobin?

a. Platelet ☐
b. Erythrocyte ☐
c. Thrombocyte ☐
d. Leukocyte ☐

58. Which of the following lab tests can be used as an indicator of dehydration?

a. BUN ☐
b. PTT (partial thromboplastin time) ☐
c. Serum potassium ☐
d. Hematocrit ☐

59. A _____ can be used to administer nutrition or long-term chemotherapy.

a. Peg tube ☐
b. Chest tube ☐
c. Venous catheter ☐
d. J-tube ☐

60. The administration of IV (intravenous) injection gadolinium (Gd) contrast media is indicated for MRI during:

a. Pediatric imaging ☐
b. Abdominal imaging ☐
c. Brain & Spine imaging ☐
d. a, b, and c ☐

61. The percent (%) of patients who have been "reported" to have had reactions to contrast agents (gadolinium) in MRI is:

a. Less than 2% ☐
b. 5% ☐
c. 15% ☐
d. 20% ☐

62. Patients who are at an "increased risk" of reactions to gadolinium include:
   1. A history of asthma and/or allergies
   2. Prior contrast reactions
   3. Hemolytic anomalies
   4. All patients

> **a.** 1 only ☐
> **b.** 1 and 2 only ☐
> **c.** 1, 2, and 3 only ☐
> **d.** 1, 2, 3, and 4 ☐

63. Patients who "have been reported" to have had reactions to gadolinium include:
   1. A history of asthma and/or allergies
   2. Prior contrast reactions
   3. Hemolytic anomalies
   4. All patients

> **a.** 1 only ☐
> **b.** 1 and 2 only ☐
> **c.** 1, 2, and 3 only ☐
> **d.** 1, 2, 3, and 4 ☐

64. Contrast agent reactions, such as flushing, hives, and nausea, are called:

> **a.** Psychosomatic ☐
> **b.** Cardiovascular ☐
> **c.** Anaphylactic ☐
> **d.** Nonsystemic ☐

65. If you determine that an adult patient needs CPR, what should be your first response?

> **a.** Call for help ☐
> **b.** Begin cardiac compressions ☐
> **c.** Begin mouth to mouth ☐
> **d.** Begin the Heimlich maneuver ☐

66. When performing one-rescuer CPR on an adult, the rate of compressions to ventilations should be:

> **a.** 5:2 ☐
> **b.** 15:2 ☐
> **c.** 15:1 ☐
> **d.** 30:2 ☐

67. What is the most severe form of convulsive seizures?

- **a.** Grand mal ☐
- **b.** Petit mal ☐
- **c.** Epileptic ☐
- **d.** Partial ☐

68. If CPR is not started within _____ of cardiac arrest, there will be brain damage due to lack of oxygen.

- **a.** 1–3 minutes ☐
- **b.** 4–6 minutes ☐
- **c.** 7–10 minutes ☐
- **d.** 15 minutes ☐

69. Which type of shock is caused by failure of the heart to pump enough blood to the vital organs?

- **a.** Hypovolemic shock ☐
- **b.** Septic shock ☐
- **c.** Anaphylactic shock ☐
- **d.** Cardiogenic shock ☐

70. When lifting a patient, what must one remember?
- **1.** Keep your back straight
- **2.** Keep your arms straight
- **3.** Keep your knees slightly bent

- **a.** 1 only ☐
- **b.** 2 only ☐
- **c.** 1 and 3 only ☐
- **d.** 1, 2, and 3 ☐

71. Log rolling is a method of moving patients with a suspected:

- **a.** Head injury ☐
- **b.** Vertebral column injury ☐
- **c.** Extremity fracture ☐
- **d.** Bowel obstruction ☐

72. The most common site(s) injured by technologists while caring for patients is(are) the:

- **a.** Head ☐
- **b.** Arms and shoulders ☐
- **c.** Lumbosacral spine ☐
- **d.** Lower leg ☐

73. During the movement and transfer of patients, urinary catheter bags should be placed:

> **a.** Below the level of the MR couch ☐
> **b.** At the foot end of the MR couch ☐
> **c.** Below the level of the urinary bladder ☐
> **d.** On the stretcher on the sheet with the patient ☐

74. When venipuncture is performed:

> **a.** The technologist is not responsible for obtaining patient history because the exam was ordered by a physician. ☐
> **b.** The contrast agent should NEVER be flushed through the syringe, any tubing used, and the needle before injection ☐
> **c.** The contrast agent must be cooled to make it easier to inject ☐
> **d.** The contrast agent must ALWAYS be flushed through the syringe, any tubing used, and needle before injection to avoid the administration of air into the vein ☐

75. Which of the following may cause a patient to experience a syncopal episode?
  1. Hypertension
  2. Anxiety
  3. Infection
  4. Hunger

> **a.** 1 and 2 only ☐
> **b.** 1 and 3 only ☐
> **c.** 2 and 3 only ☐
> **d.** 2 and 4 only ☐

76. The diabetic patient who has excessive insulin in their body is said to have:

> **a.** Hypotension ☐
> **b.** Hyperglycemia ☐
> **c.** Hypoglycemia ☐
> **d.** Hyperkalemia ☐

77. If a patient has a cardiac arrest during MR imaging, the technologist should:

> **a.** Call a code and direct them to the scan room ☐
> **b.** Quench the magnet ☐
> **c.** Begin CPR while the patient remains within the MR scan room ☐
> **d.** Begin CPR while transferring the patient out of the scan room ☐

78. During any emergency that occurs during MR imaging, the technologist should:

> **a.** Call a code and direct the team to the scan room ☐
> **b.** Quench the magnet ☐
> **c.** Continue imaging and call the radiologist ☐
> **d.** Remove the patient from the MR scan room ☐

79. A patient experiencing tachycardia will have a:

> **a.** Slow respiratory rate ☐
> **b.** Rapid pulse rate ☐
> **c.** Low oxygen saturation reading ☐
> **d.** High blood pressure reading ☐

80. What is the average pulse rate for an infant?

> **a.** 40–60 beats per minute ☐
> **b.** 70–80 beats per minute ☐
> **c.** 80–100 beats per minute ☐
> **d.** 115–130 beats per minute ☐

81. A normal blood pressure for an adult is:

> **a.** 80/120 mmHg ☐
> **b.** 120/80 mmHg ☐
> **c.** 250/120 mmHg ☐
> **d.** 120/250 mmHg ☐

82. Which of the following blood pressure readings would indicate shock?

> **a.** Diastolic pressure of 40 mmHg ☐
> **b.** Diastolic pressure of 90 mmHg ☐
> **c.** Systolic pressure of 100 mmHg ☐
> **d.** Systolic pressure of 160 mmHg ☐

83. A patient receiving oxygen should NOT have temperature measured via the _____ route.

> **a.** Axillary ☐
> **b.** Rectal ☐
> **c.** Oral ☐
> **d.** Tympanic ☐

84. A patient with epistaxis has a(n):

a. Nose bleed ☐
b. Ear infection ☐
c. Slow pulse rate ☐
d. Abscess ☐

85. Shock resulting from large loss of body fluid or blood is called:

a. Cardiogenic ☐
b. Septic ☐
c. Hypovolemic ☐
d. Neurogenic ☐

86. For an unconscious patient who has sustained a head injury, the main concern is:

a. Preventing additional hemorrhage ☐
b. Keeping a patent airway ☐
c. Maintaining a normal pulse rate ☐
d. Maintaining adequate oxygenation ☐

87. Geriatric patients likely exhibit all EXCEPT which of the following?

a. Changes in anatomic landmarks ☐
b. Fragile skin ☐
c. Decrease in intelligence ☐
d. Difficulty with balance ☐

88. A technologist may administer oxygen in an emergency situation. The most frequent rate used is:

a. 2 L/min ☐
b. 5 L/min ☐
c. 10 L/min ☐
d. 15 L/min ☐

89. The artery that is typically used to check an adult's pulse rate is the:

a. Apical ☐
b. Carotid ☐
c. Femoral ☐
d. Radial ☐

90. The pulse used to check for circulation during CPR in an adult is the:

a. Apical ☐
b. Carotid ☐
c. Femoral ☐
d. Radial ☐

91. Which of the following conditions is common in a patient with COPD?

a. Bradycardia ☐
b. Orthopnea ☐
c. Dysphagia ☐
d. Epistaxis ☐

92. In order to reduce the possibility of orthostatic hypotension, the technologist should:

a. Sit the patient up slowly from the recumbent position and allow sufficient time sitting before proceeding to standing up ☐
b. Provide the patient with something sweet to eat or drink to counteract excess insulin in the system ☐
c. Elevate the patient's legs 60 degrees above the heart ☐
d. Place the patient in the Trendelenberg position and call for help ☐

93. Where would a "central line" catheter be located?

a. Subclavian vein ☐
b. Brachiocephalic artery ☐
c. Median cubital vein ☐
d. Superior vena cava ☐

94. A patient with apraxia will have difficulty with:

a. Speaking ☐
b. Balance ☐
c. Dressing ☐
d. Swallowing ☐

95. A patient with aphasia will have difficulty with all of the following EXCEPT:

a. Speaking ☐
b. Reading ☐
c. Dressing ☐
d. Swallowing ☐

96. Severe hypoxia has a pulse oximetry reading of:

- **a.** 95–100% ☐
- **b.** 91–94% ☐
- **c.** 86–90% ☐
- **d.** 85% and below ☐

97. An adverse reaction or event caused by treatment by a healthcare professional is called:

- **a.** Idiopathic ☐
- **b.** Nosocomial ☐
- **c.** Iatrogenic ☐
- **d.** Anaphylactic ☐

98. A normal pulse rate range for an adult is:

- **a.** 40–60 bpm ☐
- **b.** 60–90 bpm ☐
- **c.** 80–100 bpm ☐
- **d.** 100–130 bpm ☐

99. Another term used for "fever" is:

- **a.** Hyperglycemia ☐
- **b.** Hypothermia ☐
- **c.** Febrile ☐
- **d.** Dyspnea ☐

100. A patient recovering from a seizure should be:

- **a.** Placed in the recovery position (Sim's) ☐
- **b.** Instructed to lie on their back ☐
- **c.** Administered emergency oxygen ☐
- **d.** Helped to move to a more comfortable area ☐

Interpersonal communications

101. The first stage of the grieving process is:

- **a.** Anger ☐
- **b.** Denial ☐
- **c.** Depression ☐
- **d.** Bargaining ☐

102. According to Maslow's hierarchy of needs, which of the following is NOT considered to be a physiologic need?

- **a.** Food and water ☐
- **b.** Sexual fulfilment ☐
- **c.** Sleep ☐
- **d.** Morality ☐

103. The best way to validate that the patient understands correctly information presented by the technologist is to:

- **a.** Ask the patient if they understood what was said ☐
- **b.** Observe the patient nodding their head "yes" or "no" ☐
- **c.** Have the patient restate the information back to the technologist ☐
- **d.** Have the patient write down what was said ☐

104. The technologist should remain standing when explaining a procedure to a child.

- **a.** True ☐
- **b.** False ☐

105. For patients with hearing loss, each of the following would be helpful for effective communication EXCEPT:

- **a.** Avoid noisy backgrounds ☐
- **b.** Speak loudly in a high pitch ☐
- **c.** Face the patient as you speak to him/her ☐
- **d.** Rephrase what you said as necessary ☐

106. Patients with mental impairment (mental retardation/mental health issues) will better understand directions stated clearly, one at a time and in simple language. All patients with mental impairment should be presented with instructions in this manner.

- **a.** True ☐
- **b.** False ☐

107. All of the following are examples of behaviors that are likely to vary with cultural beliefs EXCEPT:

- **a.** Direct eye contact is preferred ☐
- **b.** Language spoken may differ ☐
- **c.** Ability to feel pain ☐
- **d.** Giving someone a hug to comfort them ☐

108. Which of the following is NOT a true statement regarding patients with an altered state of consciousness?

> **a.** They may not remember verbal instructions ☐
> **b.** They will not remember conversations or statements made while in an ☐
>   altered state
> **c.** It is important to continue communicating with unconscious patients ☐
> **d.** They may provide answers to questions that are incorrect or not ☐
>   pertaining to the actual question

109. It is important for children, in particular, to be given choices ONLY when a choice exists.

> **a.** True ☐
> **b.** False ☐

110. We all have what is referred to as a safe "personal space" distance. We also have a distance at which we feel safe when interacting with healthcare providers, e.g. when a procedure is being explained. The distance at which a patient will feel "safe" during such an encounter is:

> **a.** 1 foot ☐
> **b.** 3 feet ☐
> **c.** 5 feet ☐
> **d.** This distance varies for each patient ☐

Infection control

111. In which direction should the top flap of a wrapped sterile package or tray be opened?

> **a.** Toward the individual ☐
> **b.** Away from the individual ☐
> **c.** Toward the dominant hand ☐
> **d.** Away from the dominant hand ☐

112. When sterile fields are prepared, damp packages:

> **a.** Are always considered contaminated ☐
> **b.** Are always considered sterile because the dampness confirms they were ☐
>   cleaned
> **c.** Should be unwrapped first and placed in the center of the sterile field ☐
> **d.** Are always considered sterile; the dampness is only a remnant of the ☐
>   gassing process

113. A common device used for high-pressure steam sterilization is called the:

> **a.** Thermal ventilator ☐
> **b.** Vector chamber ☐
> **c.** Autoclave ☐
> **d.** Inhalator ☐

114. When the body is invaded by pathogens, what is the response in the bloodstream?

> **a.** Red blood cell count increases ☐
> **b.** White blood cell count increases ☐
> **c.** Serum count increases ☐
> **d.** Platelet count increases ☐

115. Isolation that is used for patients who have a depressed immune system is known as:

> **a.** Enteric isolation ☐
> **b.** Protective isolation ☐
> **c.** Respiratory isolation ☐
> **d.** Contact isolation ☐

116. How should linen be handled in cases of suspected salmonella contamination?

> **a.** It should be placed in a red contamination bag ☐
> **b.** It should be placed in the dirty linen as usual ☐
> **c.** It should be stored in a separate dirty linen compartment for 24 hours ☐
> **d.** It should be placed in a bag and sent to the incinerator immediately ☐

117. According to the Centers for Disease Control and Prevention (CDC), what type of isolation precautions should be used for HIV-positive patients?

> **a.** Strict ☐
> **b.** Respiratory ☐
> **c.** Enteric ☐
> **d.** Standard (universal) ☐

118. Under which of the following conditions would a sterile package NOT be considered contaminated (i.e. safe to use)?

> **a.** Package has a tear in it ☐
> **b.** Tape used to indicate sterility is intact ☐
> **c.** Package is damp ☐
> **d.** Package expiration date has been exceeded ☐

119. A sterile tray that has been set up on a table or cart will have a border of _____ that must be considered NOT sterile.

- **a.** ½ inch ☐
- **b.** 1 inch ☐
- **c.** 4 inches ☐
- **d.** 12 inches ☐

120. The process of reducing the number of possible pathogenic microorganisms by using chemical disinfectants is called:

- **a.** Sterilization ☐
- **b.** Surgical asepsis ☐
- **c.** Medical asepsis ☐
- **d.** Infection control ☐

121. An infection that is acquired in a hospital or healthcare facility is called a(n):

- **a.** Iatrogenic infection ☐
- **b.** Nosocomial infection ☐
- **c.** Idiopathic infection ☐
- **d.** Fomite infection ☐

122. Diseases, such as malaria, in which microorganisms are transferred via an insect come under the classification of _____ infections.

- **a.** Nosocomial ☐
- **b.** Indirect contact ☐
- **c.** Common vehicle ☐
- **d.** Vector borne ☐

123. Which type of blood cell is responsible for phagocytosis?

- **a.** Leukocyte ☐
- **b.** Erythrocyte ☐
- **c.** Platelet ☐
- **d.** Lymphocyte ☐

124. The source of infection where pathogens thrive in numbers sufficient to cause a threat is known as a:

    a. Carrier   ☐

    b. Droplet   ☐

    c. Reservoir   ☐

    d. Fomite   ☐

125. Which portion of a sterile surgical gown is NOT considered to be sterile?

    a. Arms   ☐

    b. Chest area   ☐

    c. Waist area   ☐

    d. Back   ☐

126. Which of the following items would NOT be a type of fomite in MRI?

    a. Head coil   ☐

    b. MRI table   ☐

    c. Syringe for injection   ☐

    d. Mouse at the control panel   ☐

127. Airborne contamination can be prevented by using special types of ventilation systems.

    a. True   ☐

    b. False   ☐

128. Droplet contamination frequently occurs via:

    a. Sneezing   ☐

    b. Shaking hands   ☐

    c. Normal breathing   ☐

    d. Sharing the operator console mouse   ☐

129. The best method to prevent the spread of microorganisms is:

    a. Handwashing   ☐

    b. Disinfecting counters and other workspaces   ☐

    c. Sterilizing as many materials as possible   ☐

    d. The inflammatory response   ☐

130. When removing personal protective apparel, which item should be removed first?

> **a.** Mask ☐
> **b.** Gown ☐
> **c.** Gloves ☐
> **d.** It does not matter in which order apparel is removed ☐

131. For droplet precautions, healthcare workers as well as visitors must wear:

> **a.** A gown only ☐
> **b.** A mask only ☐
> **c.** Gown and mask ☐
> **d.** Gown, mask, and gloves ☐

132. When cleaning, clean from:

> **a.** Bottom to top ☐
> **b.** Most contaminated area to least contaminated area ☐
> **c.** Least contaminated area to most contaminated area ☐
> **d.** The least dusty area to the most dusty area ☐

133. Disinfectants will provide a method for:

> **a.** Sterilization ☐
> **b.** Surgical asepsis ☐
> **c.** Medical asepsis ☐
> **d.** Improved body hygiene ☐

MRI screening and safety

134. Family members and ancillary personnel accompanying the patient into the scan room:

> **a.** Need not be screened because they are not undergoing MRI ☐
> **b.** Can enter the scan room to check on the patient but cannot stay during scanning ☐
> **c.** Should be screened as if they are going through the procedure themselves ☐
> **d.** Must wear a lead apron during the procedure ☐

135. In preparation for the MRI examination, patients should be encouraged to:

a. Wear their own clothing so as to feel "at home" with the study ☐
b. Wear a wrist watch so they are aware of the length of the exam ☐
c. Keep their hearing aid in so as to hear the commands and requests of ☐
   the technologist
d. Change into a hospital gown or a scrub suit provided by the imaging ☐
   center and known to be MR safe (containing no metallic components
   such as snaps and/or zippers)

136. Mrs Jones has just been sent to the MRI department from the emergency room, following a severe motor vehicle accident. She has suffered a fracture of C3 and her physicians are concerned about a cervical spinal cord compression at that level. Select the best method for proceeding with this case.

a. Rush her quickly into the scanner on her own stretcher so as not to ☐
   aggravate the fracture
b. Ask her and her family about the possibility of her having metal ☐
   fragments in her body
c. On finding out that she has had a total hip replacement, cancel the exam ☐
d. Allow her to wear her favorite gold necklace during the procedure ☐

137. Persons that should be educated about the effects of the static magnetic field, especially in high field superconducting magnets, include:
1. The nursing staff and the code team
2. The housekeeping staff and members of the fire department
3. The anesthesiologists and respiratory therapists
4. The technologist and the radiologist

a. 4 only ☐
b. 1 and 4 only ☐
c. 1,3, and 4 only ☐
d. 1, 2, 3, and 4 ☐

138. According to the White Paper on MRI safety, persons are identified into "levels" whereby "Level 2" personnel include:

a. Persons with no MRI safety training ☐
b. Persons with limited MRI safety training ☐
c. Persons with extensive training in MRI safety to include the broader ☐
   aspects of MRI (such as the magnetic field, gradient and RF fields – to
   name a few)
d. There are no Level 2 personnel in the White Paper of MRI safety ☐

139. According to the White Paper on MRI safety, imaging centers should be separated into "Zones" including all of the following EXCEPT:

a. Zone 0 – the parking lot ☐
b. Zone 1 – freely accessible to any "Level" of MR personnel ☐
c. Zone 2 – the interface between Zone 1 and Zone 3 ☐
d. Zone 3 – the "warm" Zone, generally the console area and the last stop ☐
before the scan room
e. Zone 4 – The "hot" Zone, the scan room itself ☐

140. A screening questionnaire for patients about to undergo MRI should include information about:

a. Prior injuries ☐
b. Prior surgery and implants ☐
c. Pregnancy ☐
d. All of the above ☐

141. The terminology for devices and implants in MRI was modified a few years ago, whereby the term MR compatible has been replaced with all of the following EXCEPT:

a. MR reliable ☐
b. MR safe ☐
c. MR unsafe ☐
d. MR conditional ☐

142. Absolute contraindications to MRI include:
1. Intracranial vascular clips, unless they are KNOWN to be safe
2. Cardiac pacemakers, unless they are KNOWN to be safe
3. Pregnancy
4. Intraocular, ferrous foreign bodies

a. 1 only ☐
b. 1 and 2 only ☐
c. 1, 2, and 3 only ☐
d. 1, 2, and 4 only ☐

143. The accepted standard of care for the detection of intraocular ferrous foreign bodies is:

a. Computed tomography ☐
b. MRI ☐
c. Plain film ☐
d. Visual examination ☐

144. A method that is more accurate in the detection of small intraocular ferrous foreign bodies is:

a. Computed tomography (CT) ☐
b. MRI ☐
c. Plain film ☐
d. Visual examination ☐

145. Before a patient enters the MRI environment they should be screened for:

a. Prior injuries ☐
b. Prior surgical implants ☐
c. Pregnancy ☐
d. All of the above ☐

146. Of the following implants, which would be considered acceptable to scan by MRI?

a. Ferrous aneurysms clips ☐
b. Neurostimulators ☐
c. Cardiac pacemakers ☐
d. Heart valves ☐

147. If monitoring is to be achieved by electrical and/or mechanical devices, it is important that compatibility with the MR system be demonstrated by:

a. Clearance by the FDA (Food and Drug Administration) ☐
b. Prior testing ☐
c. Manufacturer declaration ☐
d. All of the above ☐

148. The following items are usually allowed to enter the scan room in high magnetic field systems:

> **a.** Surgical stainless steel hemostats ☐
> **b.** Surgical stainless steel scissors ☐
> **c.** Copper tools ☐
> **d.** Laryngoscopes ☐

149. When used for MRI, cables from RF coils and ECG leads should be:

> **a.** Braided and placed straight through the imager ☐
> **b.** Laid along the patient's right arm, along the bore ☐
> **c.** Formed into loops within the imager ☐
> **d.** Neatly coiled and ready for use ☐

150. Surface coil cables can potentially cause damage to the patient when:

> **a.** They are not frayed and rest along the arm of the patient ☐
> **b.** They are slightly touching the patient and are frayed ☐
> **c.** They are looped and not touching the patient ☐
> **d.** All of the above ☐
> **e.** None of the above ☐

151. A quench can be used to:

> **a.** Improve image quality in MRI ☐
> **b.** Rapidly remove superconductivity and the magnetic field ☐
> **c.** Maintain magnetic field homogeneity ☐
> **d.** Satisfy the thirst of the technologist ☐
> **e.** Lubricate the magnet coils ☐

152. During a quench, patients and operators should be evacuated from the room to avoid:

> **a.** Asphyxiation and frostbite ☐
> **b.** Subarachnoid hemorrhage ☐
> **c.** Ruptured tympanic membranes ☐
> **d.** a and c ☐
> **e.** a, b, and c ☐

153. What is regulated by the FDA?

> **a.** Length of the bore ☐
> **b.** Diameter of the bore ☐
> **c.** Acoustic noise ☐
> **d.** Scan time ☐

154. For optimum operation of MRI systems, the ambient temperature and relative humidity should remain between:

> **a.** 30°F and 50°F/30% and 50% ☐
> **b.** 65°F and 75°F/50% and 70% ☐
> **c.** 70°F and 90°F/70% and 100% ☐
> **d.** No specific temperature or humidity range ☐

155. The acceptable safe level for exposure to magnetic fringe fields with respect to patients with cardiac pacemakers has been reported to be:

> **a.** Between 5 g and 15 g ☐
> **b.** Between 5 T and 15 T ☐
> **c.** Between 15 g and 30 g ☐
> **d.** Below 5 g ☐

156. Magnetic field shielding can be achieved either actively or passively. Passive shielding can be achieved by lining the MRI room with:

> **a.** Copper ☐
> **b.** Steel ☐
> **c.** Lead ☐
> **d.** None of the above ☐

157. RF shielding can be achieved by lining the MRI room with:

> **a.** Copper ☐
> **b.** Steel ☐
> **c.** Lead ☐
> **d.** None of the above ☐

158. It is acceptable for the general population to be exposed to a field strength of:

> **a.** 2.0 Tesla ☐
> **b.** 4.0 Tesla ☐
> **c.** 8.0 Tesla ☐
> **d.** 5.0 gauss ☐

159. The unit of measure of RF absorption is:

> **a.** Watts per pound ☐
> **b.** Volts per pound ☐
> **c.** Watts per kilogram ☐
> **d.** Volts per kilogram ☐

160. MR imagers are magnetic field shielded such that:

> **a.** Any metallic objects can enter the scan room ☐
> **b.** The fringe field is confined to / within the bore ☐
> **c.** The fringe field is confined to / within the scan room ☐
> **d.** There is no fringe field ☐

161. Fringe files are less of a concern for:

> **a.** Mid-field superconducting imagers ☐
> **b.** Low-field resistive imagers ☐
> **c.** High-field superconductive imagers that are shielded ☐
> **d.** Low field, vertical field permanent magnet imagers ☐

162. In July of 2003, The FDA's Center for Devices & Radiological Health (CDRH) modified the limit on RF absorption (dose) to _____ for the HEAD.

> **a.** 2.0 W/kg absorption for 5 minutes ☐
> **b.** 3.0 W/kg absorption for 10 minutes ☐
> **c.** 4.0 W/kg absorption for 15 minutes ☐
> **d.** 12.0 W/kg absorption for 5 minutes ☐

163. The Food and Drug Administration (FDA) limits the allowable RF absorption to:

> **a.** 0.2 W/kg averaged over the body ☐
> **b.** 0.4 W/kg averaged over the body ☐
> **c.** 2.0 W/kg averaged over the body ☐
> **d.** 4.0 W/kg averaged over the body ☐

164. The term used to describe RF absorption is:

a. Sensitive acquisition range (SAR) ☐
b. Specific absorption rate (SAR) ☐
c. Susceptibility attack region (SAR) ☐
d. None of the above ☐

165. The predominant biologic effect of RF fields is:

a. Induced voltages ☐
b. Tissue heating ☐
c. Hypothermia ☐
d. Magnetic hemodynamic effect ☐

166. RF antenna effects can cause:

a. Better reception on your car radio ☐
b. RF interference artifacts ☐
c. Thermal injury and flames ☐
d. b and c ☐

167. The FDA limits the effect of RF absorption to an increase in core body temperature of:

a. 0.1 °C ☐
b. 1 °C ☐
c. 10 °F ☐
d. There is no limit ☐

168. The increase in body temperature as the result of RF absorption is:

a. Barely detectable ☐
b. Greatest on the outside, becoming less at the center ☐
c. Greatest at the center, becoming less on the surface ☐
d. Evenly distributed throughout the body ☐

169. RF energy used in MRI is classified as:

a. High energy, ionizing radiation ☐
b. High energy, nonionizing radiation ☐
c. Low energy, nonionizing radiation ☐
d. Low energy, ionizing radiation ☐

170. As the flip angle is doubled, RF deposition increases by a factor of:

    a. One ☐
    b. Two ☐
    c. Three ☐
    d. Four ☐

171. RF heating is more of a concern in imaging sequences such as:

    a. Gradient echo ☐
    b. Echo planar ☐
    c. Spin echo ☐
    d. Fast spin echo ☐

172. Areas of the body that are most sensitive to the heat (from SAR) are:

    a. Brain and spinal cord ☐
    b. Vertebral bodies ☐
    c. Globes of the eyes and testicles ☐
    d. Pancreas and liver ☐

173. For adult imaging in MRI, the FDA guidelines limit the field strength of clinical imagers to:

    a. 1.5 T and below ☐
    b. 2 T and below ☐
    c. 4.0 T ☐
    d. 8.0 T ☐

174. A magnetic field strength of 1 T is equal to:

    a. 1000 g ☐
    b. 10 000 g ☐
    c. 100 000 g ☐
    d. 10 g ☐

175. All of the following are regulated by the FDA EXCEPT:

    a. Field strength of the main magnet for clinical imaging ☐
    b. RF absorption (SAR) ☐
    c. Gradient length ☐
    d. Acoustic noise ☐

176. No biologic effects have been reported in humans as the result of exposure to:

    a. Static magnetic fields above 2 T ☐
    b. Time-varying magnetic fields ☐
    c. RF fields ☐
    d. Static magnetic fields below 2 T ☐

177. The field strength at isocenter is measured in units of:

    a. Gauss ☐
    b. Tesla ☐
    c. Watts ☐
    d. SAR ☐

178. Magnetic field strength outside the imager is usually measured in:

    a. Gauss ☐
    b. Tesla ☐
    c. Watts ☐
    d. SAR ☐

179. The attractive force that an object will experience at a distance of 6 feet from isocenter is dependent on:

    a. The ferromagnetic properties of the object ☐
    b. The mass of the object ☐
    c. The field strength of the system ☐
    d. All of the above ☐

180. As a conductive medium (e.g. blood) moves across a magnetic field, an effect known as the magnetic hemodynamic effect occurs, resulting in:

    a. Increased blood pressure ☐
    b. Increased temperature ☐
    c. Elevated T-wave ☐
    d. No noticeable effect ☐

181. It is _____ for all patients to be provided with hearing protection in the form of _____.

    a. Required/headphones or earplugs ☐
    b. Recommended/headphones or earplugs ☐
    c. Required/head coil ☐
    d. Recommended/helmet ☐

182. The gradient magnetic fields:

> **a.** Produce heat in the gradient coils during the scan ☐
> **b.** Can produce noise to cause temporary hearing loss ☐
> **c.** Change rapidly during the scanning process ☐
> **d.** All of the above ☐

183. When a patient is placed within the bore of a magnetic resonance imager, an effect can be noted on the ECG whereby there is an elevated "T" wave. This "effect" is known as all EXCEPT:

> **a.** Magnetohydrodynamic effect ☐
> **b.** Magnet-hydrodynamic effect ☐
> **c.** Magnet-hemodynamic effect ☐
> **d.** Magnetophosphenes ☐

184. The "effect" whereby the patient experiences a visual impression of seeing "stars in their eyes", is known as _____.

> **a.** Magnetohydrodynamic effect ☐
> **b.** Magnet-hydrodynamic effect ☐
> **c.** Magnet-hemodynamic effect ☐
> **d.** Magnetophosphenes ☐

185. The FDA limit on time-varying magnetic fields is _____.

> **a.** 10 G/cm ☐
> **b.** 6 T/s ☐
> **c.** 1 G/cm ☐
> **d.** Until the patient experiences peripheral nerve stimulation ☐

186. Time-varying magnetic field (TVMF) effects include all of the following EXCEPT:

> **a.** Heat and increased body temperature ☐
> **b.** Acoustic damage and hearing loss ☐
> **c.** Peripheral nerve stimulation and tingling ☐
> **d.** Magnetophosphenes and "stars in the eyes" ☐

187. TVMF effects are of greater concern for which scan sequences?

a. FSE ☐
b. EPI ☐
c. GE ☐
d. SE ☐

188. The strength of gradient magnetic fields is measured in:

a. MilliTesla per meter ☐
b. Watts per kilogram of body weight ☐
c. Watts per time ☐
d. Gauss per centimeter ☐
e. a and d ☐

189. Gradient magnetic fields are a safety concern because they:

a. Produce large amounts of RF energy ☐
b. Induce currents in conductors ☐
c. Cause short-term memory loss ☐
d. All of the above ☐

190. Time-varying magnetic fields have been reported to have caused:

a. Mild cutaneous sensations and images of flashing lights in patients ☐
b. Involuntary muscle contractions and cardiac arrhythmias in patients ☐
c. Neither of the above ☐
d. a and b ☐

191. The FDA limit for the static magnetic field for clinical imaging for patients over 1 month of age is:

a. 1.0T ☐
b. 1.5T ☐
c. 4.0T ☐
d. 8.0T ☐

192. The FDA limit for the static magnetic field for clinical imaging (including any and all patients) is:

a. 1.0T ☐
b. 1.5T ☐
c. 4.0T ☐
d. 8.0T ☐

193. The imaging sequence that is of most concern for time-varying magnetic field effects is:

> **a.** Spin echo ☐
> **b.** Gradient echo ☐
> **c.** Fast spin echo ☐
> **d.** Echo planar ☐

194. Gradient rise time is:

> **a.** The time it takes for a gradient to get to full amplitude ☐
> **b.** The time it takes for the cake to rise ☐
> **c.** The time it takes for one TR to occur ☐
> **d.** The time it takes for one acquisition to be complete ☐

195. The duty cycle is:

> **a.** The time it takes for the gradient to reach its full amplitude ☐
> **b.** The time it takes for one TR to occur ☐
> **c.** The time the gradients are on during a TR period ☐
> **d.** How much the gradient changes the magnetic field over a specific ☐
> distance

196. To avoid auditory damage during MRI, all patients should be offered:

> **a.** Headphones ☐
> **b.** Earplugs ☐
> **c.** Antinoise devices ☐
> **d.** a and b ☐
> **e.** a, b, and c ☐

Part A: Answers

1. b

2. c

The plaintiff is the person (patient) bringing suit and the defendant is the person (healthcare provider) being sued.

To establish a claim of malpractice, four conditions must be proved true:

1. The defendant had a duty to provide reasonable care to the patient

2. The patient has sustained some type of loss or injury

3. The defendant is the party responsible for the loss

4. The loss is attributable to negligence or improper practice

3. c

Beneficence and nonmaleficence are two ethical terms. Beneficence is to only do good and to prevent evil or harm. It is not always possible to practice beneficence. Case in point: a needle stick is somewhat painful, yet necessary to inject IV contrast media.

4. b

There are two types of negligence: intentional and unintentional. This type of situation most likely falls under the category of unintentional negligence.

5. d

6. b

Res ipsa loquitor is a Latin term meaning "the thing speaks for itself".

7. b

8. d

9. c

Assault and battery are terms frequently linked together. Assault is threatening to cause physical harm. Battery is actually causing physical harm.

10. b

The good effect must be the only intention. In other words, the healthcare worker is not purposely causing pain, anxiety or harm. The good effect is what is intended and the bad effect is unintended or an indirect consequence.

11. a

12. c

13. b

Tort law encompasses recovery of damages for a civil wrong for which the law provides a remedy. Tort action is filed to recover damages for personal injury or property damage occurring from negligent conduct or intentional misconduct.

14. d

15. b

The patient must understand in laymen's terms (or terms that said patient can understand) what will happen during the procedure. The patient does not need to know every single little detail regarding the procedure.

16. c

17. d

18. c

19. b

Invasion of privacy is also a breach of confidentiality. Only those parties with a need to know should be privy to this type of confidential information.

20. a

21. b

It is not within the MRI technologist's scope of practice to provide the patient with a diagnosis. Questions regarding diagnosis and treatment must be referred to the physician.

22. b

23. b

24. b

25. c

26. b

27. a

28. d

ARRT Standard of Ethics 2011

Statement of purpose

The purpose of the ethics requirements is to identify individuals who have internalized a set of professional values that cause one to act in the best interests of patients. This internalization of professional values and the resulting behavior is one element of ARRT's definition of what it means to be qualified. Exhibiting certain behaviors as documented in the Standards of Ethics is evidence of the possible lack of appropriate professional values.

The Standards of Ethics provides proactive guidance on what it means to be qualified and to motivate and promote a culture of ethical behavior within the profession. The ethics requirements support the ARRT's mission of promoting high standards of patient care by removing or restricting the use of the credential by those who exhibit behavior inconsistent with the requirements. www.arrt.org

Code of Ethics

The Code of Ethics forms the first part of the Standards of Ethics. The Code of Ethics shall serve as a guide by which Certificate Holders and Candidates may evaluate their professional conduct as it relates to patients, healthcare consumers, employers, colleagues, and other members of the healthcare team. The Code of Ethics is intended to assist Certificate Holders and Candidates in maintaining a high level of ethical conduct and in providing for the protection, safety, and comfort of patients. The Code of Ethics is aspirational.

1. The radiologic technologist acts in a professional manner, responds to patient needs, and supports colleagues and associates in providing quality patient care.
2. The radiologic technologist acts to advance the principal objective of the profession to provide services to humanity with full respect for the dignity of mankind.
3. The radiologic technologist delivers patient care and service unrestricted by the concerns of personal attributes or the nature of the disease or illness, and without discrimination on the basis of sex, race, creed, religion, or socio-economic status.
4. The radiologic technologist practices technology founded upon theoretical knowledge and concepts, uses equipment and accessories consistent with the purposes for which they were designed, and employs procedures and techniques appropriately.
5. The radiologic technologist assesses situations; exercises care, discretion, and judgment; assumes responsibility for professional decisions; and acts in the best interest of the patient.
6. The radiologic technologist acts as an agent through observation and communication to obtain pertinent information for the physician to aid in the diagnosis and treatment of the patient and recognizes that interpretation and diagnosis are outside the scope of practice for the profession.
7. The radiologic technologist uses equipment and accessories, employs techniques and procedures, performs services in accordance with an accepted standard of practice, and demonstrates expertise in minimizing radiation exposure to the patient, self, and other members of the healthcare team.
8. The radiologic technologist practices ethical conduct appropriate to the profession and protects the patient's right to quality radiologic technology care.
9. The radiologic technologist respects confidences entrusted in the course of professional practice, respects the patient's right to privacy, and reveals confidential information only as required by law or to protect the welfare of the individual or the community.
10. The radiologic technologist continually strives to improve knowledge and skills by participating in continuing education and professional activities, sharing knowledge with colleagues, and investigating new aspects of professional practice.

Rules of Ethics

The Rules of Ethics form the second part of the Standards of Ethics. They are mandatory standards of minimally acceptable professional conduct for all Certificate Holders and Candidates. Certification and Registration are methods of assuring the medical community and the public that an individual is qualified to practice within the profession. Because the public relies on certificates and registrations issued by ARRT, it is essential that Certificate Holders and Candidates act consistently with these Rules of Ethics. These Rules of Ethics are intended to promote the protection, safety, and comfort of patients. The Rules of Ethics are enforceable. Certificate Holders and Candidates engaging in any of the following conduct or activities, or who permit the occurrence of the following conduct or activities with respect to them, have violated the Rules of Ethics and are subject to sanctions as described hereunder. www.arrt.org

It is always recommended to review the most current version of this, or any document "quoted" within this book.

29. a

Although there are times when colleagues need to discuss the clinical situation, this particular scenario requires no discussion among colleagues. When a request is clearly incorrect (e.g. the patient injures the knee, but imaging of the shoulder is ordered), the technologists needs to contact the referring physician to correct the order. In this case, no further discussion is required.

30. c

A syncopal episode means that the patient has fainted. Patients who are nervous (anxiety) and/or hungry (possibly hypoglycemic) are more likely to faint.

31. d

There are patients who do require medication (sedation) to enable them to complete the MR examination. If medication has not been ordered prior to the MR examination, the study may need to be rescheduled. However, most patients can endure the procedure when handled "delicately".

32. d

All such patients should be monitored in MRI because verbal communication with them can be difficult. This has been recommended by the Safety Committee for the ISMRM (International Society for Magnetic Resonance in Medicine) and also the ACR (American College of Radiology). White Paper on MRI Safety www.acr.org

33. a

Diazepam (brand name Valium) is a respiratory depressant, so respiratory monitoring should be considered with such patients.

34. a

The Safety Committee for the SMR states in its guidelines and recommendations for monitoring of patients in MRI that: "It is good practice for all patients that undergo MRI to be visually and/or verbally monitored."

35. a

BEFORE 2010, package inserts for all FDA-approved gadolinium chelates listed "No Known" contraindications. As of 2010, the ACR produced a MRI Safety Manual for Contrast Media, known as the Contrast Media Update. It was observed in 2007, that the administration of gadolinium to patients with renal insufficiency (or acute renal injury) can cause a deadly condition known as NSF (nephrogenic systemic fibrosis). For this reason as of 2010, contrast media is contraindicated in patients with known renal impairment, acute renal injury or renal function of below 30. The glomerular filtration rate (GFR) is calculated from the patient's creatinine, age, race, and sex.

36. c

37. d

38. c

At this time, only one agent has been approved for pediatric and abdominal imaging. All have been approved for central nervous system imaging. Technically, gadolinium is NOT FDA approved for intra-articular injection. However, since gadolinium is commonly injected intra-articularly, it has become the "accepted standard of care".

39. c

Hypoglycemia is a condition whereby the diabetic patient does not have enough sugar in the system for the insulin delivered to metabolize. A diabetic patient who does not have enough insulin and has too much sugar in the body would experience hyperglycemia.

40. a

41. d

Since the MRI table (or couch) is not capable of "tilting" into the Trendelenberg position, the legs can be elevated 60' (degrees) to achieve the same result.

42. c

Ice is preferred to heat for contrast extravasation. The ice localizes the area of fluid collection, keeping it from spreading to more tissue and causing damage to those tissues. Extravasation must ALWAYS be documented. In moderate to severe extravasation, the referring physician must be notified. Check and follow institutional policies for extravasation.

43. b

IV solution should be kept at a height of 18 −20 inches above the vein. Solution higher than this will run too fast, possibly causing extravasation. Solution lower than this height can lead to the back flow of blood.

44. c

Superficial veins are used for contrast media injections. Common veins to use are often found in the antecubital area of the arm: cephalic, accessory cephalic, antecubital and basilic. Remember to avoid using the arm on the same side as a mastectomy site or the affected side for a stroke patient. Also avoid areas of scarring, burns, and bruising.

45. b

Although it can be used for multiple doses, the multidose vial should ONLY be used for one patient.

46. a

47. c

48. d

Routine blood tests performed to assess renal function (prior to contrast administration for imaging studies) are: serum creatinine and blood urea nitrogen (BUN)

49. b

Hematocrit is a blood test that can be used to detect dehydration. When administration of contrast media is anticipated, it is best that the patient be well hydrated in order to more efficiently excrete the contrast media via the kidneys.

50. a

The tunica media is the middle layer of an artery or vein. It is the elastic, muscular layer. It is thicker in an artery due to the increased pressure of blood flow versus venous return.

51. b

Lab results should be reported for each patient along with a normal range for that particular facility. Normal ranges may vary somewhat between facilities. Creatinine is an indicator of renal function. Creatinine is a by-product of creatine. Creatine is related to muscle function. Therefore, creatinine (and creatine) varies with the amount of muscle within the body. So, for example, a young male body builder could have a creatinine of 2.0 within the bloodstream; this could be "normal" for this particular patient. However, the same creatinine level in an older female patient (who is light in weight with little muscle mass) would be high. Therefore, the creatinine is only an *indicator* of renal function. For this reason, the GFR (glomerular filtration rate) or eGFR (estimated glomerular filtration rate) should be calculated to evaluate renal function prior to the administration of gadolinium.

52. d

53. c

54. a

The pulmonary arteries carry deoxygenated blood from the right ventricle to the lungs for oxygenation. The oxygenated blood then returns to the left atrium via the pulmonary veins.

55. a

The outer layer of the artery or vein can be called either the tunica adventitia or tunica externa.

56. c

57. b

An erythrocyte is a red blood cell.

58. d

59. c

60. d

61. a

62. b

63. d

Although any patient can react to gadolinium (or any medication including saline), patients with allergies and asthma (and/or those who have previous history of reactions) do have a higher risk of reacting. Bear in mind that any (or all) patient(s) can have serious anaphylactic reactions (and death) from the administration of contrast.

64. d

Systemic refers to the entire body (being affected). Nonsystemic refers to only a portion of the body (being affected). Flushing and hives occur only in a particular portion of the body at one time; therefore they are nonsystemic responses.

65. a

An adult requiring CPR most likely needs to be defibrillated; a physician or qualified nurse trained in the use of the defibrillator, which should be on the crash cart, is required. This situation refers to a healthcare setting where crash carts with defibrillators are routinely found. (Not to a defibrillator that can be used by the general public.)

66. d

67. a

68. a

69. d

70. c

71. b

72. c

Proper body mechanics for moving patients should always be observed. Use the legs (slightly apart for balance) with knees slightly bent, instead of the back. It is also better to push than to pull with the arms.

73. c

Urinary catheters are often a cause of nosocomial urinary tract infections. One reason for this is due to the backflow of urine into the bladder associated with NOT keeping the urine collection bag below the level of the bladder.

74. d

75. d

A syncopal episode means that the patient has fainted. Patients who are nervous (anxiety) and/or hungry (possibly hypoglycemic) are more likely to faint.

76. c

Hypoglycemia is a condition whereby the diabetic patient does not have enough sugar in the system for the insulin delivered to metabolize. A diabetic patient who does not have enough insulin and has too much sugar in the body would experience hyperglycemia.

77. d

The White Paper on MRI Safety, published by the blue ribbon panel of MRI experts, recommends that the patient be removed from the scan room and, if possible, resuscitation procedures begun. For more information about MRI safety, visit the ACR website www.acr.org to obtain the most current version of the Safety documents. Also, information can be found on the MRI safety website www.mrisafety.com

78. d

Regardless of the nature of the emergency, it is always prudent to remove the patient out of the magnetic field, such that intervention can be safely administered.

79. b

80. d

81. b

Blood pressure measurements indicate the "pressure" of blood flow during systole (while the heart is in contraction) and diastole (while the heart is in relaxation). In a normal adult, a systolic pressure of 120 and a diastolic pressure of 80 are considered to be normal values. Although both systolic and diastolic pressures are important factors, when the diastolic pressure increases (even up to 90), this is considered mild hypertension (or high blood pressure) since the heart should be in its relaxation phase.

82. a

83. c

The oral route should also not be used for patients who are mouth breathers (and who have just had a warm or cold drink or meal). Taking a rectal temperature may cause stimulation of the vagus nerve, which may cause additional problems for patients with certain cardiac conditions. Rectal temperature is considered to be the most accurate and axillary the least accurate.

84. a

85. c

86. b

A "patent" airway refers to an open airway.

87. c

88. a

Oxygen is considered a medication and as such must be prescribed by a physician. In an emergency, the technologist may administer oxygen. The rate of 1–4 L/minute is considered a safe amount to administer via nasal cannula or a regular face mask. Rates of 5 L/minute or higher must be administered using a type of humidification system to avoid excessive drying out of mucosal membranes.

89. d

90. b

The carotid pulse is found over the carotid artery toward the anterolateral aspect of the neck. The carotid bifurcation is located at the level of C-3 (at the angle of the mandible). The radial pulse, found in the wrist over the radial artery at the base of the thumb, is the pulse used in "routine" circumstances. To remember the location of the radial artery and ulnar artery (in the wrist) the radial is on the thumb side; "R-T".

91. b

Orthopnea means that the patient has difficulty breathing when lying down. This is a common problem in patients with COPD (emphysema).

92. a

Orthostatic hypotension is abnormally low blood pressure resulting from standing up too fast after lying down. This happens most often in elderly patients and can result in the patient fainting. The technologist should allow ample time for the patient to sit, allowing blood pressure to return to normal.

93. a

94. c

Apraxia can occur after a "brain injury" such as a stroke. Apraxia is the inability to perform "learned motor skills". These patients understand directions, but are unable to complete a task, such as getting dressed.

95. c

Aphasia can occur after a "brain injury" such as a stroke. Aphasia is the inability to complete language tasks such as speaking, reading and writing. These patients may have receptive aphasia (wherein they cannot understand what is being said to them) or expressive aphasia (wherein they can understand what is being said but cannot respond appropriately). In addition, aphasic patients can have difficulty swallowing.

96. d

At 85% oxygenation or less, body organs will not receive enough oxygen to support their needs and functions. They may experience ischemia and eventually infarction or necrosis if left untreated.

97. c

Iatrogenic, by definition means: "Of or relating to illness caused by medical examination or treatment." by dictionary.com.

98. b

99. c

Febrile is defined as pertaining to or marked by fever; feverish (dictionary.com). A febrile seizure (or convulsion) is a seizure caused by a high fever.

100. a

In the recovery position (Sim's), the patient is lying on their left side, semi-prone with the upper leg bent for support, so that the mouth is turned downward. This will prevent aspiration of any fluid (or vomitus) that may be draining from the mouth.

101. b

The five stages of grieving (in order), according to Elizabeth Kubler-Ross, are: denial, anger, bargaining, depression, and acceptance.

102. d

103. c

104. b

It is best to be on the same level with children to avoid intimidating them. This is true for all patients (such as a patient in a wheel chair).

105. b

Most hearing loss is in the higher pitch or range. For this reason, speaking in a low pitch and speaking very slowly will help the patient who is hearing impaired to understand your directions.

106. a

Patients with any type of mental impairment will significantly vary in their ability to understand and comply with directions. Each patient must be evaluated on an individual basis and treated accordingly with respect.

107. c

Many perceptions, behaviors, actions, and interpretations depend on cultural beliefs. This applies not only to patients and their families, but to our coworkers as well. It is important to keep in mind that variations also exist within each culture. It is beneficial to become familiar with cultural differences, while avoiding stereotyping.

108. b

109. a

Choose your words carefully in these situations. Example: Do NOT ask a young child if they "want to get up onto the table for you"; tell them that you need them to get up onto the table. Examples of a viable choice might be – which bandage do you want? or which sticker would you like? This same logic holds true for patients who are mentally impaired, but each patient needs to be assessed on an individual basis. Be careful when providing adults with choices as well.

110. d

Personal space is a very variable distance from one person to another. Cultural beliefs also play a huge role in perception of how close one person should come to another in any situation. It is our responsibility as technologists to determine what makes a patient feel comfortable. When touching a patient is necessary as part of what we are doing, we need to take the time to explain what we are about to do and always to use a professional, firm, appropriate touch.

111. b

112. a

113. c
Items that have the potential to rust should not be sterilized in an autoclave.

114. b

115. b

116. a

117. d
Follow standard precautions for ALL patients at ALL times for safety and infection control.

118. b
Packaging or any sterile item that becomes damp prior to use is NOT considered sterile. The moisture invites microorganisms to collect in that area. Tape or labels that indicate sterility vary from one institution to another. This method of verifying sterility is often used when items are sterilized "in house". The technologist must be familiar with institutional procedures and protocols regarding sterilization.

119. b
The one-inch area border (or edges) of the sterile tray is NOT considered sterile since those edges are most likely to come in contact with a nonsterile item or person. When pouring a solution into a cup on a sterile tray, the bottle of solution may leak or drip toward the bottom of the bottle, causing an area of dampness.

120. c
Surgical asepsis is the process of sterilization, which will eliminate microorganisms and their spores.

121. b

122. d

123. a
A leukocyte is a white blood cell. Phagocytosis occurs when microorganisms enter the body and fluids carrying white blood cells travel to the site to destroy them.

124. c

125. d
The area under the arms (or the armpits) is not considered sterile due to dampness caused by perspiration.

126. c
A fomite is an object that carries microorganisms from one person to another via indirect contact.

127. a

Airborne contamination occurs via transmission of dust particles or droplets that have evaporated and contain infectious microorganisms. Special ventilation systems reduce the number of particles and droplets.

128. a

Droplets can be spread by sneezing, coughing, and speaking, and depositing the droplets into the mucous membranes of the face. Droplets travel short distances of 3 feet or less and do not remain suspended in air.

129. a

130. c

For a gown tied in the front, the ties should be unfastened first. Next, gloves are removed (using proper technique). Hands should then be washed. The mask is removed next using only the ties (the mask itself is considered contaminated). Remove the gown in the proper manner. Always wash your hands again.

131. b

132. c

133. c

134. c

135. d

136. b

137. d

In addition to patients, system operators, and hospital staff, the fire department and housekeeping personnel might also inadvertently enter the scan room with ferromagnetic materials. For this reason, such persons should be educated.

138. c

The White Paper on MRI safety states that there are levels of "expertise" associated with MRI safety whereby:
- Non-MR personnel have little or no training in MRI safety
- Level 1 personnel have limited training in MRI safety (education about the magnetic field)
- Level 2 personnel have extensive training in MRI safety, including training in not only the magnetic field but also the RF and gradient fields, and their safety considerations

139. a

The White Paper on MRI safety recommends that imaging centers are separated into "Zones" whereby:
- Zone 1 – freely accessible to any "Level" of MR personnel; can include the parking lot
- Zone 2 – the interface between Zone 1 and Zone 3; generally the reception area

- Zone 3 – the "warm" Zone, generally the console area and the last stop before the scan room. It is recommended that there is a lock between Zone 2 and Zone 3 to avoid someone inadvertently wandering into the scan room
- Zone 4 – the "hot" Zone; the scan room itself

140. d

In many cases information about prior injuries, surgery, and/or pregnancy can identify those patients who may require consideration for MRI imaging (What protocol should be performed? Should contrast be administered? Should the patient be scanned at all?).

141. a

The term MR compatible has been replaced with the following terms:
- MR safe – this device can ALWAYS be scanned (or brought into the scan room) at any time, in any field strength, with NO restrictions.
- MR unsafe – this device can NEVER be scanned (or brought into the scan room) at any time, in any field strength.
- MR conditional – this device MIGHT be scanned (or brought into the scan room) with specific restrictions (or under specific conditions).

142. d

Since the 1990s, intracranial vascular clips have been made of MR conditional metals (including titanium). These clips are MR conditional and can be scanned under certain "conditions". As of 2011, a new pacemaker was developed to be MR conditional. This "pacing system" can be imaged under particular "conditions".

143. c

Studies have shown that intraocular ferrous foreign bodies (IFFB; metallic fragments) that are smaller than can be detected by the resolution of plain film radiography are too small to cause ocular damage. For this reason, even though CT is more sensitive to the presence of metallic fragments, the standard of care for the detection of IFFB is plain film radiography – including two views (Waters view + lateral) and/or (Waters view with eyeballs looking upwards and again looking downwards).

144. a

145. d

146. d

147. d

The Safety Committee for the Society for Magnetic Resonance (SMR) has published a statement to this effect in its guidelines and recommendations for monitoring of patients in MRI.

148. c

Many surgical supplies are extremely magnetic and should not enter the scan room of high-field systems until they have been tested and proven safe.

149. a

150. d

Even though cables may look to be in excellent condition, any cable loops within the imager can potentially receive induced voltages. Therefore, cables that touch the patient are automatically looped, given that the human body is conductive and the patient completes the loop.

151. b

152. d

During a quench, asphyxiation can result from the loss of oxygen, frostbite from the low temperatures of cryogens, and ruptured tympanic membranes from the increased pressure in the scan room that occurs as the liquid cryogen (He) returns to gas.

153. c

154. b

Relatively low temperatures and humidities enable optimal use of MRI systems.

155. d

156. b

157. a

158. d

The FDA limit for clinical imaging, with respect to field strength, used to be 2.0T. As of July 2003, the regulations were changed whereby the FDA limit was increased to 4.0T for all patients and 8.0T for children aged 1 month and older. To answer this question, one must realize that the patients who are scheduled for MR imaging are screened prior to entering the scan room to avoid any contraindicated materials from entering with them, and hence the high magnetic field. When evaluating the "general population", one should assume that these persons have NOT been screened and could potentially possess contraindicated devices. For this reason, the "general population" should be restricted to within 5.0 Gauss.

159. c

160. c

There is a fringe field concern even for superconductive imagers that are magnetic field shielded. Shielding is used to confine the fringe field. The MR imager that is of "lesser" concern from the fringe field is the low field, vertical field, permanent magnet.

161. d

The FDA/CDRH modified the regulations in July of 2003 to absorption of RF (dose) averaged over the whole body and/or RF absorption that varies with anatomic location. In addition, the amount of RF is also measured by time of exposure. The regulations are:

Site	Dose	Time (min)	SAR > (W/kg)
• Whole body	Averaged over	15	4
• Head	Averaged over	10	3
• Head or torso	Per gram of tissue	5	8
• Extremities	Per gram of tissue	5	12

162. c

163. d

164. b

165. b
RF effects include increase in body temperature due to tissue heating. (Induced voltages come from gradients. Magnet hemodynamic effects come from the static magnetic field. Hypothermia results from exposure to cryogens during a quench.)

166. d
Voltages induced in RF coils can cause heat and, possibly, flames, and/or artifacts on MR images

167. b

168. b

169. c

170. d

171. d
Because fast spin echo uses a train (determined by the echo train length) of RF pulses to fill several lines of k-space per TR and acquire images faster, tissue heating increases with increased RF. As flip angle increases, RF power deposition increases. As flip angle doubles (from 90 degrees to 180 degrees) RF power increases by a factor of 4 (four).

172. c

173. d

174. b

175. c
The FDA (Food and Drug Administration) has regulations that monitor any, and all, devices for the safety and efficacy of that device. The components of the MR system that the FDA has specific guidelines include:
1. The static magnetic field
    a. The FDA limit for clinical imaging is 4.0T (Tesla) for all patients
    b. The FDA limit for clinical imaging is 8.0T (Tesla) for patients over one month of age.
2. The RF absorption

    a. Measured in SAR (Specific Absorption Rate)

    b. The FDA limit for SAR = 4.0 watts / kilogram

    c. The FDA also limits RF by anatomic location

3. Magnetic field gradients (also known as time-varing magnetic fields – TVMF)

    a. TVMF causes peripheral nerve stimulation

        i. The FDA limit for TVMF, used to be 6 Tesla per second (T/s)

            1. T/s is expressed in units of dB/dt

            2. The equation... dB/dt = dV .defines Faraday's law of induction

                a. dB – a change magnetic field

                b. dt – a change in time

                c. dV – a change in voltage

            3. When a magnet moves (dB) near a conductor (in this case, the human body), there is a voltage (dV) created within the conductor (manifesting as peripheral nerve stimulation, PNS).

            4. The amount of voltage (dV) or PNS is related to the strength of the magnet b and the rate at which it moves (dt).

        ii. In July of 2003, The FDA's Center for Devices & Radiological Health (CDRH) modified the limit on gradients (TVMF)

        iii. The FDA/CDRH limit for TVMF is "Until the patient feels painful nerve stimulation"

    b. Since the gradients produce acoustic noise, another TVMF affect is acoustic noise

        i. The US FDA limit for sound is140 dB (decibels) or 99 dB with hearing protection in place [USFDA 2003]

    c. Gradient characteristics

        i. Gradient strength is expressed in milliTesla per meter (mT/M) or Gauss per centimeter (g/cm).

        ii. Gradient speed or rise time is expressed in microseconds (μs)

        iii. The combination of rise time and strength is expressed as the Slew rate and is expressed in units of Tesla per meter per second (T/M/s)

        iv. The length of the gradient is not a factor in TVMF effects, and therefore is NOT FDA regulated. www.acr.org

176. d

177. b

178. a

179. d

The more ferromagnetic, the greater the mass, and the stronger the magnetic field, the greater the attractive force.

180. c

This can be noticed in patients who are monitored with ECG leads and enter the bore of the imager.

181. b

182. d

183. d

Faraday's Law of induction states that if a conductor moves through a magnetic field, a voltage is induced within the conductor. In this case, as blood flows through the magnetic field (blood being a conductor) a voltage is induced and displayed onto the ECG monitor. This effect is known as the Magnet-hemodynamic effect and/or the Magnet-hydrodynamic effect and/or the Magnetohydrodynamic effect.

184. d

Faraday's law of induction states that if a conductor moves through a magnetic field, a voltage is induced within the conductor. In this case, as the gradient fields are switched on and off during image acquisition, a voltage is induced within the retinal phosphenes. The result is a phenomenon known as magnetophosphenes, whereby the patient experiences the sensation of "stars in their eyes".

185. d

186. a

187. b

188. e

Gradient strength is measured in field strength over distance (mT/m or G/cm) whereby $10\,mT/m = 1\,g/cm$.

189. b

190. d

191. c

192. c

The FDA has changed the limit for field strength for clinical imaging from, up to 2.0T, to 4.0T for infants (up to 1 month of age) and 8.0T for patients over one month of age.

193. d

Echo planar imaging uses gradients with very rapid rise times because all of the K space is filled in one TR time by changing the amplitude of the gradient as many as 128, 256 or 512 times per TR period.

194. a

195. c

196. e

Some companies do offer antinoise devices for MRI systems. However, earplugs can reduce noise by 10–20 dB and this is sufficient to reduce auditory effects in MRI.

Part B

Imaging Procedures

Clinical Applications, Enhancement Agents, Cross-Sectional Anatomy

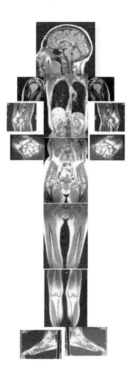

Introduction

Although imaging protocols vary with facility, there are a number of aspects of clinical imaging that are universal. Despite slight procedural variations, the fundamental components are basically the same, including T1-weighted images (usually acquired to evaluate anatomy) and T2-weighted images (usually acquired for pathology). Also, when small anatomy is to be imaged, high-resolution imaging is required [small field of view (FOV), thin slice thickness, and/or high imaging matrix]. Such fundamental parameters are of importance to most practicing technologists.

MRI procedure questions make up roughly 30% of the examination.

Part B offers review questions that pertain to cross-sectional anatomy, physiology, clinical imaging (including parameters and options, coil selection, positioning, and landmark), and contrast enhancement (dose, administration, effects on the image).

Review Questions for MRI, Second Edition. Carolyn Kaut Roth and William H. Faulkner.
© 2013 Carolyn Kaut Roth and William S. Faulkner. Published 2013 by Blackwell Publishing Ltd.

Type of study	Focus of questions

1. Head and Neck
  a. Brain
  b. Internal auditory canal
  c. Pituitary
  d. Orbit
  e. Soft tissue neck
  f. Angiography
  g. Spectroscopy
  h. fMRI
2. Spine
  a. Cervical
  b. Thoracic
  c. Lumbo-sacral
3. Thorax
  a. Brachial plexus
  b. Cardiac
  c. Breast
  d. Mediastinum
  e. Angiography
4. Abdomen
  a. Liver, spleen, pancreas
  b. Kidneys, adrenals
  c. Peritoneum, retroperitoneum
  d. Biliary
  e. Angiography
5. Pelvis
  a. Female pelvis
  b. Male pelvis
6. Musculoskeletal
  a. Temporo-mandibular joint (TMJ)
  b. Upper extremities
    • Shoulder
    • Elbow
    • Wrist
    • Hand
  c. Lower extremities
    • Hip
    • Knee
    • Ankle
    • Foot
	Questions about each of the studies listed on the left may focus on any of the following factors:
	1. Anatomy and physiology
	  • Imaging planes
	  • Pathological considerations
	  • Protocol considerations
	2. Contrast
	  • Type of agent (FDA approved)
	  • Contraindications
	  • Dose calculation
	  • Administration route
	  • Effects on image
	3. Patient positioning
	  • Coil selection and position
	  • Patient orientation
	  • Centering and landmark
	  • Physiologic gating and triggering

MRI of the head and neck

Although protocols vary from site to site, there are general protocols that are used for brain imaging in MRI. A typical brain protocol includes: three-plane localizer (or scout), sagittal T1WI, axial T2WI, axial FLAIR imaging, and diffusion imaging. If the patient is imaged for "specialized" imaging of the head [such as the internal auditory canals (IACs) or pituitary], high resolution would be acquired for the visualization of smaller structures associated with the pituitary gland and/or within the IACs.

Questions 1–137 concern the head and neck.

MRI of the spine

MRI spine protocols vary from site to site, but there are general protocols that are used for spine imaging in MRI. A typical spine protocol includes: three-plane localizer (or scout), sagittal T1WI (high resolution), sagittal T2WI (high resolution), axial T1 and T2*, and 3D gradient echo imaging. If the patient is imaged for "specialized" imaging of the spine, contrast-enhanced imaging would be acquired for the visualization of enhancing lesions and/or the postoperative lumbar spine.

Questions 138–194 concern the spine.

MRI of the thorax

MRI thorax (chest, heart, vasculature, and breast) protocols vary from site to site, but there are general protocols that are used for thorax imaging in MRI. A typical thorax protocol includes: three-plane localizer (or scout), coronal T1WI (high resolution), axial T1 and T2, and 3D gradient echo imaging (with contrast enhancement for vasculature and breast lesions).

Questions 195–285 concern the thorax.

MRI of the abdomen and pelvis

MRI abdomen protocols vary from site to site, but there are general protocols that are used for abdomen imaging in MRI. A typical abdomen protocol includes: three-plane localizer (or scout), coronal T1WI or T2W axial T2WI, and axial T1W gradient echo imaging acquired in-phase and out-of-phase. Additional abdominal imaging includes 3D gradient echo imaging (with contrast enhancement for visceral and/or vasculature lesions). Most abdominal imaging is acquired with breath-hold rapid imaging and/or respiratory triggering techniques to reduce the motion artifact caused by breathing.

Questions 286–435 concern the anatomy and imaging procedures for visceral structures, including the liver, spleen, pancreas, kidneys, adrenals, stomach, and bowel.

MRI of the musculoskeletal system

MRI musculoskeletal protocols vary from site to site, but there are general protocols that are used for musculoskeletal imaging in MRI. A typical musculoskeletal protocol includes: three-plane localizer (or scout) and three planes (sagittal, axial, coronal – to the plane of the joint acquired with oblique imaging) acquired with both T1 and T2 contrast. Also, most facilities will acquire a STIR sequence in the plane that best demonstrates the anatomy and/or pathology of interest.

Questions 436–596 concern the anatomy and imaging procedures for musculoskeletal structures, including the temporo-mandibular joint (TMJ), shoulder, elbow, wrist, hand, hip, knee, ankle, and foot.

Part B: Questions

MRI of the head and neck

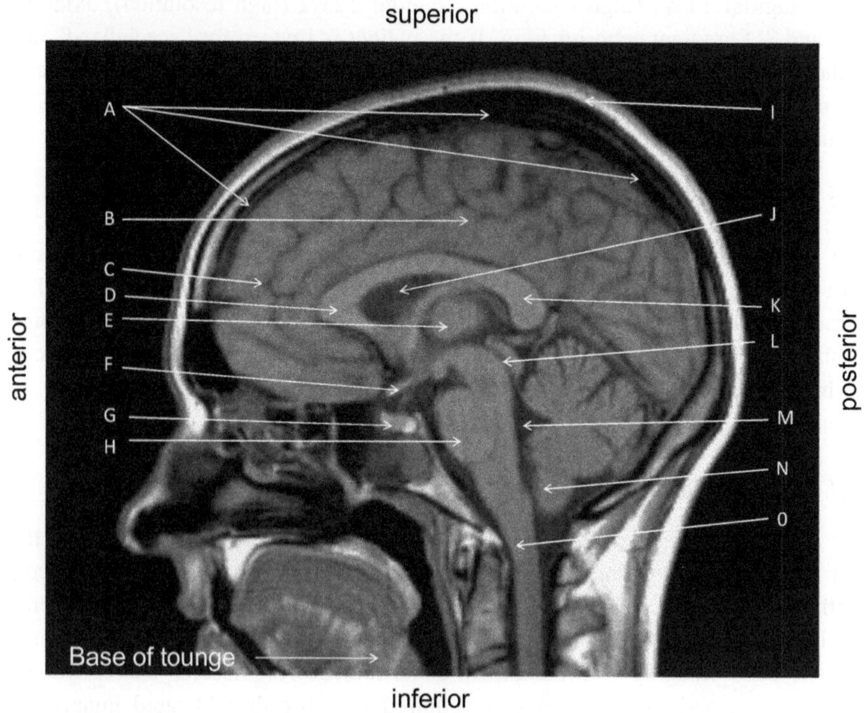

Figure B.1

1. Figure B.1 was acquired in the:

   a. Axial imaging plane ☐
   b. Sagittal imaging plane ☐
   c. Coronal imaging plane ☐
   d. Off-axis (oblique) imaging plane ☐

2. Figure B.1 is an example of a:

   a. T1-weighted image ☐
   b. T2-weighted image ☐
   c. Spin (proton) density-weighted image ☐
   d. T2*-weighted image ☐
   e. None of the above ☐

3. Figure B.1 is likely to be acquired with:

> **a.** Short TR and short TE ☐
> **b.** Short TR and Long TE ☐
> **c.** Long TR and Long TE ☐
> **d.** Long TR and short TE ☐

4. On Figure B.1 arrow A is pointing to the:

> **a.** Cerebrospinal fluid (CSF) ☐
> **b.** Subcutaneous fat ☐
> **c.** Superior sagittal sinus ☐
> **d.** Frontal sinus ☐

5. On Figure B.1 the tissue indicated by arrow A is made up primarily of:

> **a.** White matter ☐
> **b.** Gray matter ☐
> **c.** Cerebrospinal fluid (CSF) ☐
> **d.** Flowing blood ☐

6. On Figure B.1 arrow B is pointing to the:

> **a.** Frontal lobe ☐
> **b.** Parietal lobe ☐
> **c.** Occipital lobe ☐
> **d.** Temporal lobe ☐

7. On Figure B.1 the tissue indicated by arrow B is made up primarily of:

> **a.** White matter ☐
> **b.** Gray matter ☐
> **c.** Cerebrospinal fluid (CSF) ☐
> **d.** Bone ☐

8. On Figure B.1 arrow C is pointing to the:

> **a.** Parietal lobe ☐
> **b.** Frontal lobe ☐
> **c.** Internal auditory canals ☐
> **d.** Fourth ventricle ☐

9. Figure B.1 arrow D is pointing to the:

a. Caudate nucleus ☐
b. Genu of the corpus callosum ☐
c. Internal capsule ☐
d. Pituitary gland ☐

10. On Figure B.1 the tissue indicated by arrow D is made up primarily of:

a. White matter ☐
b. Gray matter ☐
c. Cerebrospinal fluid (CSF) ☐
d. Bone ☐

11. On Figure B.1 arrow E is pointing to the:

a. Thalamus ☐
b. Corpus callosum ☐
c. Lentiform nucleus ☐
d. Pituitary stalk (infundibulum) ☐

12. On Figure B.1 arrow F is pointing to the:

a. Pituitary stalk ☐
b. Infundibulum ☐
c. Optic chiasm ☐
d. Optic nerve ☐

13. On Figure B.1 arrow G is pointing to the:

a. Pituitary gland ☐
b. Pineal gland ☐
c. Thalamus ☐
d. Lentiform nucleus ☐

14. On Figure B.1 arrow H is pointing to the:

a. Medulla oblongata ☐
b. Pons ☐
c. Spinal cord ☐
d. Midbrain ☐

15. On Figure B.1 arrow H is pointing to a structure that is one component of the brainstem. The components that make up the brainstem include the:

> **a.** Hypothalamus, hyperthalamus, and right and left thalamus ☐
> **b.** Caudate nucleus, lentiform nucleus, and thalamus (right and left) ☐
> **c.** Pons, medulla, and midbrain (cerebral peduncles) ☐
> **d.** Anterior cerebral arteries (right and left), posterior cerebral arteries (right and left), anterior communicating artery, and posterior communicating arteries (right and left) ☐

16. The components that make up the basil ganglia include the:

> **a.** Hypothalamus, hyperthalamus and right and left thalamus ☐
> **b.** Caudate nucleus, lentiform nucleus, and thalamus (right and left) ☐
> **c.** Pons, medulla, and midbrain (cerebral peduncles) ☐
> **d.** Anterior cerebral arteries (right and left), posterior cerebral arteries (right and left), anterior communicating artery, and posterior communicating arteries (right and left) ☐

17. The components that make up the circle of Willis include the:

> **a.** Hypothalamus, hyperthalamus, and right and left thalamus ☐
> **b.** Caudate nucleus, lentiform nucleus, and thalamus (right and left) ☐
> **c.** Pons, medulla, and midbrain (cerebral peduncles) ☐
> **d.** Anterior cerebral arteries (right and left), posterior cerebral arteries (right and left), anterior communicating artery, and posterior communicating arteries (right and left) ☐

18. The components that make up the diencephalon include the:

> **a.** Hypothalamus, hyperthalamus, and right and left thalamus ☐
> **b.** Caudate nucleus, lentiform nucleus, and thalamus (right and left) ☐
> **c.** Pons, medulla, and midbrain (cerebral peduncles) ☐
> **d.** Anterior cerebral arteries (right and left), posterior cerebral arteries (right and left), anterior communicating artery, and posterior communicating arteries (right and left) ☐

19. On Figure B.1 arrow I is pointing to the:

> **a.** Skull ☐
> **b.** Cerebrospinal fluid (CSF) ☐
> **c.** Subcutaneous fat ☐
> **d.** Meninges ☐

20. On Figure B.1 arrow J is pointing to the:

> **a.** Anterior (frontal) horn of the lateral ventricle ☐
> **b.** Posterior (occipital) horn of the lateral ventricle ☐
> **c.** Third ventricle ☐
> **d.** Fourth ventricle ☐

21. On Figure B.1 the tissue indicated by arrow J is made up primarily of:

> **a.** White matter ☐
> **b.** Gray matter ☐
> **c.** Cerebrospinal fluid (CSF) ☐
> **d.** Flowing blood ☐

22. On Figure B.1 arrow K is pointing to the:

> **a.** Genu of the corpus callosum ☐
> **b.** Body of the corpus callosum ☐
> **c.** Splenium of the corpus callosum ☐
> **d.** Choroid plexus ☐

23. On Figure B.1 arrow L is pointing to the:

> **a.** Anterior horn of the lateral ventricle ☐
> **b.** Posterior horn of the lateral ventricle ☐
> **c.** Cerebral aqueduct ☐
> **d.** Third ventricle ☐

24. On Figure B.1 the tissue indicated by arrow L is made up primarily of:

> **a.** White matter ☐
> **b.** Gray matter ☐
> **c.** Cerebrospinal fluid (CSF) ☐
> **d.** Bone ☐

25. On Figure B.1 arrow M is pointing to the:

> **a.** Anterior horn of the lateral ventricle ☐
> **b.** Posterior horn of the lateral ventricle ☐
> **c.** Third ventricle ☐
> **d.** Fourth ventricle ☐

26. On Figure B.1 the tissue indicated by arrow M is made up primarily of:

   a. White matter   ☐
   b. Gray matter   ☐
   c. Cerebrospinal fluid (CSF)   ☐
   d. Bone   ☐

27. On Figure B.1 arrow N is pointing to the:

   a. Frontal lobe   ☐
   b. Parietal lobe   ☐
   c. Occipital lobe   ☐
   d. Cerebellar tonsils   ☐

28. On Figure B.1 arrow O is pointing to the:

   a. Medulla oblongata   ☐
   b. Pons   ☐
   c. Spinal cord   ☐
   d. Midbrain   ☐

29. On Figure B.1 the tissue indicated by arrow O is made up primarily of:

   a. White matter   ☐
   b. Gray matter   ☐
   c. Cerebrospinal fluid (CSF)   ☐
   d. Bone   ☐

30. It is likely that Figure B.1 was acquired with a:

   a. Body transmit/receive coil   ☐
   b. Head transmit/receive coil   ☐
   c. 5-inch round local or surface receive-only coil   ☐
   d. Endorectal coil   ☐

31. The best view for the base of the tongue and the epiglottis is the:

a. Coronal ☐
b. Oblique ☐
c. Sagittal ☐
d. Axial ☐

32. To optimize brain imaging when evaluating patients for metastatic disease, an FDA-approved contrast agent can be administered:

a. With single dose followed by rapid imaging ☐
b. With a triple dose followed by rapid imaging ☐
c. With single dose and imaging followed by twice the dose again after ☐
30 minutes
d. a and b ☐

33. The patient with a history of seizures can be imaged using cardiac gating:

a. To minimize pulsatile flow motion artifact in the temporal lobes ☐
b. To monitor the patient for potential seizures ☐
c. To avoid talking to the patient throughout the study ☐
d. To make vessels appear black ☐

34. The best view to evaluate patients with seizures is:

a. Sagittal ☐
b. Axial ☐
c. Coronal ☐
d. Sagittal oblique ☐

35. When a patient arrives at the imaging center with a cranial scar, the technologist should:

a. Immediately perform the MRI scan to find out what surgery they
underwent ☐
b. Screen the patient, their doctor, and/or family to find out what type of
surgery they have had ☐
c. Ignore the scar ☐
d. Cover the head with a sterile drape ☐

36. When scanning patients to rule out brain tumors, the weighted images acquired to evaluate the extent of the lesion, after injection of gadolinium, are:

    a. T1 ☐
    b. T2 ☐
    c. Proton density ☐
    d. T2* gradient echo ☐

37. When imaging a patient with decreased consciousness, an area of high signal intensity is noted on both the T1- and T2-weighted images. The type of lesion is likely to be:

    a. A metastatic lesion ☐
    b. An abscess ☐
    c. A hemorrhage (methemoglobin) ☐
    d. A neurofibroma ☐

38. To best visualize the pituitary gland in MRI, the optimal planes for high-resolution T1-weighted images are:

    a. Sagittal and coronal ☐
    b. Coronal and axial ☐
    c. Axial and sagittal ☐
    d. Sagittal, axial, and coronal ☐

39. For a patient with a suspected pituitary microadenoma, contrast is injected and imaging is performed:

    a. Rapidly because lesions enhance early ☐
    b. Rapidly because lesions have low signal intensity compared to the enhanced pituitary gland ☐
    c. With delayed imaging because lesions enhance slowly and the pituitary gland does not enhance ☐
    d. With no specific timing considerations ☐

40. The optimal plane(s) for high-resolution T1-weighted images of the internal auditory canals (IACs) include:
  1. Sagittal
  2. Axial
  3. Coronal
  4. Oblique

  a. 1 and 3 only ☐
  b. 2 and 3 only ☐
  c. 1 and 2 only ☐
  d. 1, 2, 3, and 4 ☐

41. When imaging the brain of a child under 1 year of age (since the brain is not fully developed or myelinated), the BEST visualization of gray and white matter differences is demonstrated on_____, whereby white matter is hyperintense to gray matter.

  a. T1-weighted spin echo ☐
  b. T2-weighted spin echo ☐
  c. Spoiled gradient echo ☐
  d. Inversion recovery ☐

42. Typical brain protocols consist of:
  1. Sagittal T1-weighted spin echo (SE)
  2. Axial T2-weighted fast spin echo (FSE)
  3. Axial spoiled gradient echo (GrE)
  4. Axial FLAIR images or axial PDWI
  5. Coronal T2-weighted FSE
  6. Axial diffusion

  a. 1, 2, and 3 only ☐
  b. 1, 2, and 4 only ☐
  c. 1, 2, 4, and 6 only ☐
  d. 1, 2, 3, 4, 5, and 6 ☐

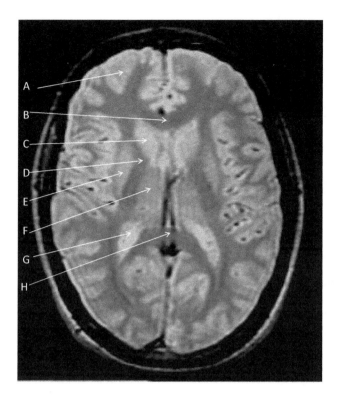

Figure B.2

43. Figure B.2 was acquired in the:

   a. Axial imaging plane ☐
   b. Sagittal imaging plane ☐
   c. Coronal imaging plane ☐
   d. Off-axis (oblique) imaging plane ☐

44. Figure B.2 is an example of a:

   a. T1-weighted image ☐
   b. T2-weighted image ☐
   c. Spin (proton) density-weighted image ☐
   d. T2*-weighted image ☐
   e. All of the above ☐

45. On Figure B.2 arrow A is pointing to the:

> **a.** Corpus callosum ☐
> **b.** Caudate nucleus ☐
> **c.** Cerebral cortex ☐
> **d.** Lateral ventricle ☐

46. On Figure B.2 arrow A is pointing to a structure composed of tissue made up primarily of:

> **a.** White matter ☐
> **b.** Gray matter ☐
> **c.** Cerebrospinal fluid (CSF) ☐
> **d.** Muscle ☐

47. On Figure B.2 arrow B is pointing to the:

> **a.** Genu of the corpus callosum ☐
> **b.** Body of the corpus callosum ☐
> **c.** Splenium of the corpus callosum ☐
> **d.** Lateral ventricle ☐

48. On Figure B.2 the structure indicated by arrow B is composed of tissue made up primarily of:

> **a.** White matter ☐
> **b.** Gray matter ☐
> **c.** Cerebrospinal fluid (CSF) ☐
> **d.** Muscle ☐

49. On Figure B.2 arrow C is pointing to the:

> **a.** Caudate nucleus ☐
> **b.** Lentiform nucleus ☐
> **c.** Internal capsule ☐
> **d.** Claustrum ☐

50. On Figure B.2 the structure indicated by arrow C is composed of tissue made up primarily of:

> **a.** White matter ☐
> **b.** Gray matter ☐
> **c.** Cerebrospinal fluid (CSF) ☐
> **d.** Muscle ☐

51. On Figure B.2 arrow D is pointing to the:

> **a.** Caudate nucleus ☐
> **b.** Lentiform nucleus ☐
> **c.** Internal capsule ☐
> **d.** Claustrum ☐

52. On Figure B.2 the structure indicated by arrow D is composed of tissue made up primarily of:

> **a.** White matter ☐
> **b.** Gray matter ☐
> **c.** Cerebrospinal fluid (CSF) ☐
> **d.** Muscle ☐

53. It is likely that Figure B.2 was acquired with a:

> **a.** Short TR and short TE ☐
> **b.** Long TR and long TE ☐
> **c.** Short TR and long TE ☐
> **d.** Long TR and short TE ☐

54. On Figure B.2 arrow E is pointing to the:

> **a.** Caudate nucleus ☐
> **b.** Lentiform nucleus ☐
> **c.** Internal capsule ☐
> **d.** Claustrum ☐

55. On Figure B.2 arrow F is pointing to the:

> **a.** Caudate nucleus ☐
> **b.** Lentiform nucleus ☐
> **c.** Internal capsule ☐
> **d.** Thalamus ☐

56. On Figure B.2 arrow G is pointing to the:

> **a.** Right, anterior (frontal) horn of the lateral ventricle ☐
> **b.** Left, anterior (frontal)horn of the lateral ventricle ☐
> **c.** Left, posterior (occipital) horn of the lateral ventricle ☐
> **d.** Right, posterior (occipital) horn of the lateral ventricle ☐

57. On Figure B.2 arrow H is pointing to the:

a. Genu of the corpus callosum ☐
b. Body of the corpus callosum ☐
c. Splenium of the corpus callosum ☐
d. Lateral ventricle ☐

58. On short TR/TE spin echo (or fast spin echo) imaging sequences, white matter appears:

a. Hyperintense to gray matter ☐
b. Hypointense to gray matter ☐
c. Hypointense to CSF ☐
d. Isointense to gray matter ☐

59. The cranial nerves running through the internal auditory canals are:

a. IV and V ☐
b. V and VI ☐
c. VI and VII ☐
d. VII and VIII ☐
e. VIII and IX ☐

60. The ACR guidelines for brain imaging suggest that the minimum imaging procedure should include a three-plane localizer (or scout) image and:

1. Sagittal T1WI
2. Axial T2WI
3. Axial PDWI and/or axial FLAIR
4. Axial T1WI pre and post gadolinium
5. Coronal T1WI
6. Diffusion imaging

a. 1, 2, 3, 4, and 5 ☐
b. 1, 2, 4, and 6 ☐
c. 1, 2, 3, and 6 ☐
d. 1, 2, 3, 4, 5, and 6 ☐

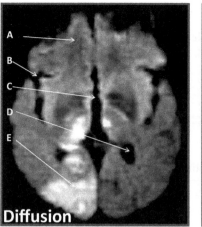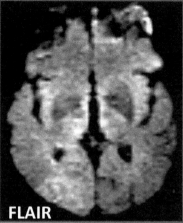

Figure B.3

61. The images in Figure B.3 were acquired in the:

    a. Axial imaging plane □
    b. Sagittal imaging plane □
    c. Coronal imaging plane □
    d. Off-axis (oblique) imaging plane □

62. Typical diffusion images (Figure B.3) are typically acquired with a B-value of:

    a. 4000 ms □
    b. 100 ms □
    c. 2200 ms □
    d. 1000 ms □

63. On Figure B.3 (left) arrow A is pointing to the:

    a. Sylvian fissure □
    b. Lateral fissure □
    c. Middle cerebral artery □
    d. Frontal lobe of the brain □

64. On Figure B.3 (left) arrow B is pointing to a structure known as ALL of the following EXCEPT the:

    a. Sylvian fissure □
    b. Lateral fissure □
    c. Middle cerebral artery □
    d. Frontal lobe of the brain □

65. On Figure B.3 (left) the arrow C is pointing to the:

a. Frontal horn of the lateral ventricle ☐
b. Posterior horn of the lateral ventricle ☐
c. Temporal horn of the ventricle ☐
d. Third ventricle ☐
e. Fourth ventricle ☐

66. On Figure B.3 (left) arrow D is pointing to the:

a. Frontal horn of the lateral ventricle ☐
b. Posterior horn of the lateral ventricle ☐
c. Temporal horn of the ventricle ☐
d. Third ventricle ☐
e. Fourth ventricle ☐

67. On a typical diffusion image (Figure B.3, left), the high signal indicated by arrow E represents:

a. Chronic infarct ☐
b. Old stroke ☐
c. Transient ischemic attack (TIA) ☐
d. Early (hyperacute) infarct ☐

68. On Figure B.3 high signal in the right posterior portion of the brain is visualized on the diffusion image (left) but not the FLAIR image (right) because:

a. Old stroke has a high fluid content ☐
b. Old stroke has unrestricted molecular diffusion ☐
c. New stroke has restricted molecular diffusion ☐
d. New stroke demonstrates T2 shine through ☐

69. For most brain imaging procedures, the patient is positioned _____ and centered for landmark at the_____.

a. Prone/acantho-meatal line ☐
b. Supine/nasion ☐
c. Supine/external auditory meatus ☐
d. None of the above ☐

70. For the evaluation of a patient with "tinnitus" images should be "centered" at the level of the:

    a. Submento-vertex ☐

    b. Nasion ☐

    c. Glabella ☐

    d. External auditory meatus (EAM) ☐

71. For optimal imaging of the thyroid gland, patients are positioned:

    a. Supine and the head coil is pulled all the way down over the neck ☐

    b. Supine and local coils are placed on the anterior neck ☐

    c. Supine and the body coil is used to ensure large FOV ☐

    d. Prone and local coils are placed on the posterior neck ☐

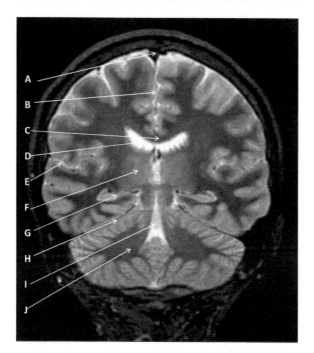

Figure B.4

72. Figure B.4 was acquired in the:

    a. Axial imaging plane ☐

    b. Sagittal imaging plane ☐

    c. Coronal imaging plane ☐

    d. Off-axis (oblique) imaging plane ☐

73. Figure B.4 is an example of a:

- **a.** T1-weighted image ☐
- **b.** T2-weighted image ☐
- **c.** Spin (proton) density-weighted image ☐
- **d.** T2*-weighted image ☐
- **e.** All of the above ☐

74. Figure B.4 was likely acquired with a spin echo or fast spin echo acquisition with a:

- **a.** Short TR and short TE ☐
- **b.** Short TR and long TE ☐
- **c.** Long TR and long TE ☐
- **d.** Long TR and short TE ☐

75. On Figure B.4 arrow A is pointing to the:

- **a.** Superior sagittal sinus ☐
- **b.** Inferior sagittal sinus ☐
- **c.** Straight sinus ☐
- **d.** Transverse sinus ☐

76. On Figure B.4 arrow B is pointing to a:

- **a.** Longitudinal fissure ☐
- **b.** Sylvian fissure ☐
- **c.** Lateral fissure ☐
- **d.** Tentorium ☐

77. On Figure B.4 arrow C is pointing to the:

- **a.** Genu of the corpus callosum ☐
- **b.** Body of the corpus callosum ☐
- **c.** Splenium of the corpus callosum ☐
- **d.** Lateral ventricle ☐

78. On Figure B.4 arrow D is pointing to the:

- **a.** Right, anterior (frontal) horn of the lateral ventricle ☐
- **b.** Left, anterior (frontal) horn of the lateral ventricle ☐
- **c.** Left, posterior (occipital) horn of the lateral ventricle ☐
- **d.** Right, posterior (occipital) horn of the lateral ventricle ☐

79. On Figure B.4 arrow E is pointing to a:

- **a.** Longitudinal fissure ☐
- **b.** Sylvian fissure ☐
- **c.** Lateral fissure ☐
- **d.** b and c ☐

80. On Figure B.4 arrow F is pointing to the:

- **a.** Frontal lobe ☐
- **b.** Parietal lobe ☐
- **c.** Thalamus ☐
- **d.** Occipital lobe ☐

81. On Figure B.4 arrow G is pointing to the:

- **a.** Frontal lobe ☐
- **b.** Parietal lobe ☐
- **c.** Temporal lobe (hippocampus) ☐
- **d.** Occipital lobe ☐

82. On Figure B.4 arrow H is pointing to a:

- **a.** Longitudinal fissure ☐
- **b.** Sylvian fissure ☐
- **c.** Lateral fissure ☐
- **d.** Tentorium ☐

83. On Figure B.4 arrow I is pointing to the:

- **a.** Right, anterior (frontal) horn of the lateral ventricle ☐
- **b.** Left, anterior (frontal) horn of the lateral ventricle ☐
- **c.** Third ventricle ☐
- **d.** Fourth ventricle ☐

84. On Figure B.4 arrow J is pointing to the:

- **a.** Frontal lobe ☐
- **b.** Parietal lobe ☐
- **c.** Occipital lobe ☐
- **d.** Cerebellum ☐

85. On Figure B.4 the CSF appears bright because:

    a. Water has a short T2 relaxation time ☐

    b. Water has a long T2 relaxation time ☐

    c. Water has a short T1 relaxation time ☐

    d. Water has a high proton density ☐

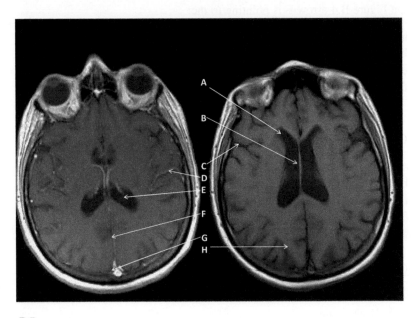

Figure B.5

86. The difference between the images demonstrated in Figure B.5 is the:

    a. Image on the left is a fat suppressed image ☐

    b. Image on the right is a fat suppressed image ☐

    c. Image on the left shows gadolinium enhancement ☐

    d. Image on the right shows gadolinium enhancement ☐

87. Gadolinium contrast media (gadolinium) provides images whereby enhancing structures (e.g. vessels or lesions) appear _____ on T1-weighted images.

    a. Hyperintense ☐

    b. Hypointense ☐

    c. Isointense ☐

    d. Dark ☐

88. Tissues with short T1 relaxation times (like fat and gadolinium = enhancing structures) appear _____ as compared to normal structures on T1-weighted images.

    a. Hyperintense/brighter than ☐
    b. Hypointense/darker than ☐
    c. Isointense/the same signal intensity as ☐
    d. Dark ☐

89. Dynamic susceptibility-weighted imaging (DCWI) is performed for the evaluation of stroke. T2* MR images are acquired before, during and after the administration of gadolinium, to provide images whereby normal brain appears _____ to brain effected by stroke.

    a. Hyperintense ☐
    b. Hypointense ☐
    c. Isointense ☐
    d. Dark ☐

90. Figure B.5 was likely to have been acquired with a spin echo (or fast spin echo) sequence using:

    a. Long TR/long TE ☐
    b. Long TR/short TE ☐
    c. Short TR/short TE ☐
    d. Short TR/long TE ☐

91. Figure B.5 was acquired in the:

    a. Axial imaging plane ☐
    b. Sagittal imaging plane ☐
    c. Coronal imaging plane ☐
    d. Off-axis (oblique) imaging plane ☐

92. On Figure B.5 arrow A is pointing to the:

    a. Anterior (frontal) horn of the lateral ventricle ☐
    b. Posterior (occipital) horn of the lateral ventricle ☐
    c. Third ventricle ☐
    d. Fourth ventricle ☐

93. On Figure B.5 the tissue indicated by arrow A is made up primarily of:

a. White matter ☐
b. Gray matter ☐
c. Cerebrospinal fluid (CSF) ☐
d. Bone ☐

94. On Figure B.5arrow B is pointing to the:

a. Septum pellucidum ☐
b. Lateral ventricle ☐
c. Sylvian fissure ☐
d. Lateral fissure ☐
e. c and d ☐

95. On Figure B.5 arrow C is pointing to the :

a. Septum pellucidum ☐
b. Lateral ventricle ☐
c. Sylvian fissure ☐
d. Lateral fissure ☐
e. c and d ☐

96. On Figure B.5 arrow D is pointing to the:

a. Right, anterior cerebral arteries ☐
b. Left, posterior cerebral arteries ☐
c. Left, lacunar branches of the middle cerebral artery ☐
d. Right, basilar artery ☐

97. On Figure B.5 arrow E is pointing to the:

a. Right, anterior (frontal) horn of the lateral ventricle ☐
b. Left, posterior (occipital) horn of the lateral ventricle ☐
c. Third ventricle ☐
d. Fourth ventricle ☐

98. On Figure B.5 arrow F is pointing to the:

a. Septum pellucidum ☐
b. Falx cerebri ☐
c. Falx cerebellari ☐
d. Choroid plexus ☐

99. On Figure B.5 arrow G is pointing to the:

a. Superior sagittal sinus ☐
b. Inferior sagittal sinus ☐
c. Transverse sinus ☐
d. Sigmoid sinus ☐

100. On Figure B.5 arrow H is pointing to the:

a. Frontal lobe ☐
b. Parietal lobe ☐
c. Temporal lobe ☐
d. Occipital lobe ☐

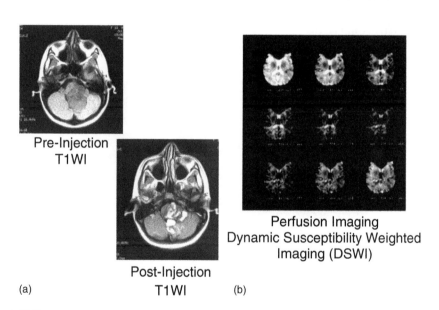

Pre-Injection
T1WI

Post-Injection
T1WI

Perfusion Imaging
Dynamic Susceptibility Weighted
Imaging (DSWI)

(a)   (b)

Figure B.6

101. The MR images in Figure B.6a are displayed without and with contrast media. The images are T1WI without and with contrast. The lesion on the enhanced image appears bright because gadolinium:

a. Shortens the T1 relaxation time ☐
b. Increases (lengthens) the T1 relaxation time ☐
c. Shortens the T2 relaxation time ☐
d. Increases (lengthens) the T2 relaxation time ☐

102. The series of nine T2* images (Figure B.6b) are EPI gradient echo sequence acquired before (upper left), during and after the administration of contrast (bottom right). The brain tissue on the enhanced image appears darker because gadolinium:

a. Shortens the T1 relaxation time ☐
b. Increases (lengthens) the T1 relaxation time ☐
c. Shortens the T2 (and T2*) relaxation times ☐
d. Increases (lengthens) the T2 (and T2*) relaxation times ☐

103. The decreased myelination found in brains of children under 1 year old results in a lack of image contrast. Consequently, in comparison to scanning adults, to achieve T2-weighted images during pediatric brain imaging often requires a:

a. Longer TE ☐
b. Longer TR ☐
c. Longer TI ☐
d. Higher flip angle ☐

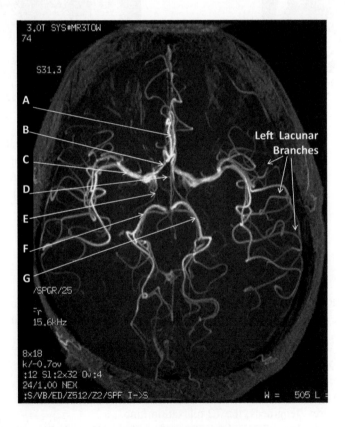

Figure B.7

104. When performing an MRA of the cerebral arteries, a saturation band should be placed _____ to axial slices:

    a. Anterior ☐
    b. Posterior ☐
    c. Superior ☐
    d. Inferior ☐

105. Figure B.7 is projected in the:

    a. Axial imaging plane ☐
    b. Sagittal imaging plane ☐
    c. Coronal imaging plane ☐
    d. Off-axis (oblique) imaging plane ☐

106. Acquired by magnetic resonance angiography (MRA), Figure B.7 is an example of a:

    a. Reformatted image ☐
    b. Segmented image ☐
    c. Collapsed image ☐
    d. Contrast-enhanced image ☐

107. On Figure B.7 arrow A is pointing to the:

    a. Right anterior cerebral artery ☐
    b. Left anterior cerebral artery ☐
    c. Right middle cerebral artery ☐
    d. Left middle cerebral artery ☐

108. On Figure B.7 arrow B is pointing to the:

    a. Right anterior cerebral artery ☐
    b. Left anterior cerebral artery ☐
    c. Right middle cerebral artery ☐
    d. Left middle cerebral artery ☐

109. On Figure B.7 arrow C is pointing to the:

    a. Right anterior cerebral artery ☐
    b. Left anterior cerebral artery ☐
    c. Right middle cerebral artery ☐
    d. Left middle cerebral artery ☐

110. On Figure B.7 arrow D is pointing to the:

> **a.** Posterior communicating artery ☐
> **b.** Middle cerebral artery ☐
> **c.** Vertebral basilar artery ☐
> **d.** Anterior cerebral artery ☐
> **e.** Anterior communicating artery ☐

111. On Figure B.7 arrow E is pointing to the:

> **a.** Posterior communicating artery ☐
> **b.** Middle cerebral artery ☐
> **c.** Vertebral basilar artery ☐
> **d.** Anterior cerebral artery ☐
> **e.** Anterior communicating artery ☐

112. On Figure B.7 arrow F is pointing to the:

> **a.** Right anterior cerebral artery ☐
> **b.** Left anterior cerebral artery ☐
> **c.** Right posterior cerebral artery ☐
> **d.** Left posterior cerebral artery ☐

113. On Figure B.7 arrow G is pointing to the:

> **a.** Right anterior cerebral artery ☐
> **b.** Left anterior cerebral artery ☐
> **c.** Right posterior cerebral artery ☐
> **d.** Left posterior cerebral artery ☐

114. When using MRA to evaluate intracranial vascularity, flow within smaller (high velocity blood flow) can best be demonstrated by:

> **a.** 2D time of flight MRA ☐
> **b.** 3D time of flight MRA ☐
> **c.** 3D phase contrast MRA ☐
> **d.** a and b ☐

115. When using MRA to evaluate extracranial vascular flow, such as that within carotid arteries, a recommended technique is:

a. 2D time of flight MRA ☐
b. 3D time of flight MRA ☐
c. 3D phase contrast MRA ☐
d. a and b ☐

116. When using MRA to evaluate peripheral vascular flow, such as that within the arteries of the legs, saturation pulses are:

a. Placed superior to the acquired slices ☐
b. Placed in the acquired slices ☐
c. Placed inferior to the acquired slices ☐
d. Not necessary ☐

117. The cranial nerve associated with the optic nerve is the:

a. First cranial nerve ☐
b. Second cranial nerve ☐
c. Third cranial nerve ☐
d. Vagus nerve ☐

118. The standard dose for gadolinium contrast media for imaging of the central nervous system (CNS) is:

a. 1.0 mL/kg (commonly known as cc/kg) ☐
b. 10 mL/kg (commonly known as cc/kg) ☐
c. 1 mmol/kg ☐
d. 0.1 mL/mmol (commonly known as cc/mmol) ☐

119. The MRA technique that is typically used for the evaluation of venous structures of the head is:

a. 2D TOF ☐
b. 3D TOF ☐
c. Contrast-enhanced MRA ☐
d. PC MRA ☐

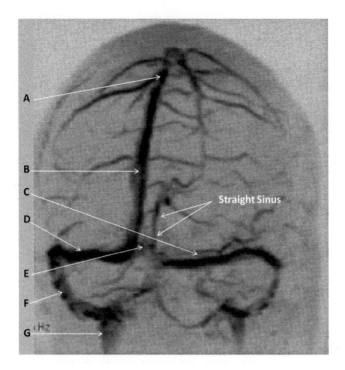

Figure B.8

120. On Figure B.8 arrow A is pointing to the:

- **a.** Right transverse sinus ☐
- **b.** Left transverse sinus ☐
- **c.** Superior sagittal sinus ☐
- **d.** Inferior sagittal sinus ☐

121. On Figure B.8 arrow B is pointing to the:

- **a.** Right transverse sinus ☐
- **b.** Left transverse sinus ☐
- **c.** Superior sagittal sinus ☐
- **d.** Inferior sagittal sinus ☐

122. On Figure B.8 arrow C is pointing to the:

- **a.** Right transverse sinus ☐
- **b.** Left transverse sinus ☐
- **c.** Superior sagittal sinus ☐
- **d.** Inferior sagittal sinus ☐

123. On Figure B.8 arrow D is pointing to the:

a. Right transverse sinus □
b. Left transverse sinus □
c. Superior sagittal sinus □
d. Inferior sagittal sinus □

124. On Figure B.8 arrow E is pointing to the:

a. Transverse sinus □
b. Superior sagittal sinus □
c. Confluence of sinuses □
d. Sigmoid sinus □
e. Internal jugular vein □

125. On Figure B.8 arrow F is pointing to the:

a. Transverse sinus □
b. Superior sagittal sinus □
c. Confluence of sinuses □
d. Sigmoid sinus □
e. Internal jugular vein □

126. On Figure B.8 arrow G is pointing to the:

a. Transverse sinus □
b. Superior sagittal sinus □
c. Confluence of sinuses □
d. Sigmoid sinus □
e. Internal jugular vein □

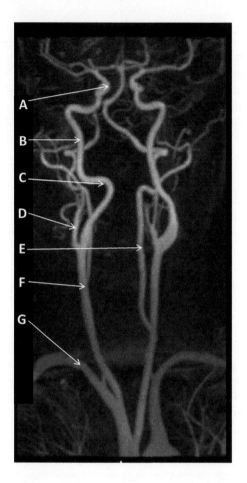

Figure B.9

127. On Figure B.9 arrow A is pointing to the:

    a. Internal carotid artery ☐
    b. External carotid artery ☐
    c. Vertebral artery ☐
    d. Subclavian artery ☐

128. On Figure B.9 arrow B is pointing to the:

    a. Internal carotid artery ☐
    b. External carotid artery ☐
    c. Vertebral artery ☐
    d. Subclavian artery ☐

129. On Figure B.9 arrow C is pointing to the:

   a. Internal carotid artery ☐
   b. External carotid artery ☐
   c. Vertebral artery ☐
   d. Subclavian artery ☐

130. On Figure B.9 arrow D is pointing to the:

   a. Internal carotid artery ☐
   b. External carotid artery ☐
   c. Vertebral artery ☐
   d. Subclavian artery ☐

131. On Figure B.9 arrow E is pointing to the:

   a. Internal carotid artery ☐
   b. External carotid artery ☐
   c. Vertebral artery ☐
   d. Subclavian artery ☐

132. On Figure B.9 arrow F is pointing to the:

   a. Internal carotid artery ☐
   b. External carotid artery ☐
   c. Common carotid artery ☐
   d. Subclavian artery ☐

133. On Figure B.9 arrow G is pointing to the:

   a. Internal carotid artery ☐
   b. External carotid artery ☐
   c. Vertebral artery ☐
   d. Subclavian artery ☐

134. The 3D contrast-enhanced MRI images of the neck vasculature shown in Figure B.9 is acquired in the:

   a. Sagittal plane ☐
   b. Axial plane ☐
   c. Coronal plane ☐
   d. Oblique plane ☐

135. On the coronal display of the neck vasculature, the vertebral arteries are located:

a. Medial to carotid arteries ☐
b. Superior to carotid arteries ☐
c. Lateral to carotid arteries ☐
d. Inferior to carotid arteries ☐

136. For optimal imaging of the thyroid gland, patients are positioned:

a. Supine and the head coil is pulled all the way down over the neck ☐
b. Supine and local coils are placed on the anterior neck ☐
c. Supine and the body coil is used to ensure a large FOV ☐
d. Prone and local coils are placed on the posterior neck ☐

137. Contrast media are utilized in CNS imaging for the evaluation of:

a. Infection ☐
b. Infarction ☐
c. Inflammation ☐
d. Neoplasm ☐
e. All of the above ☐

MRI of the spine

138. Most spine imaging is performed with the use of:

a. A surface/local coil ☐
b. ECG gating ☐
c. Respiratory compensation ☐
d. Peripheral gating ☐

139. In patients who have undergone surgery for a herniated disk in the lumbar spine, contrast enhancement can be used to distinguish recurrent disk from postoperative scar because:

a. Postoperative scar never enhances and recurrent disk does enhance ☐
b. Postoperative scar enhances and recurrent disk does not ☐
c. Disk enhances more slowly than postoperative scar ☐
d. Neither scar nor disk enhance ☐

140. For optimal imaging of the cervical spine, patient positioning and local coil placement are:

> **a.** Supine/under the neck to include from C1 to C7 ☐
> **b.** Supine/on top of the neck to include from C1 to C7 ☐
> **c.** Supine/beside the neck to include from C1 to C7 ☐
> **d.** Prone/on top of the neck to include from C1 to C7 ☐

141. On a 24-cm FOV, sagittal T-spine image that demonstrates a cord compression, the vertebral level can be determined by using:

> **a.** The xyphoid as a landmark and counting up from T12 ☐
> **b.** The sternal notch as a landmark and counting down from T1 ☐
> **c.** A large FOV localizer and counting down from C2 ☐
> **d.** Lead markers to mark T12 and T1 on large FOV images ☐

142. In lumbar spine imaging, images acquired directly through inter-vertebral disk spaces can be acquired in the:

> **a.** Axial plane ☐
> **b.** Sagittal plane ☐
> **c.** Coronal plane ☐
> **d.** Oblique plane ☐

143. On T1-weighted images of the spine, the CSF appears:

> **a.** Hyperintense to the spinal cord ☐
> **b.** Hypointense to the spinal cord ☐
> **c.** Isointense to the spinal cord ☐
> **d.** a and c ☐

144. The conus and the cauda equina in adult patients are best demonstrated by any of the following EXCEPT:

> **a.** Sagittal image of the cervical spine ☐
> **b.** Sagittal image of the thoracic spine ☐
> **c.** Sagittal image of the lumbar spine ☐
> **d.** Coronal image of the thoracic spine ☐

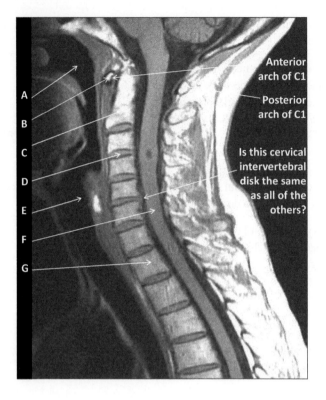

Figure B.10

145. Figure B.10 was acquired in the:

    a. Axial imaging plane ☐
    b. Sagittal imaging plane ☐
    c. Coronal imaging plane ☐
    d. Off-axis (oblique) imaging plane ☐

146. Figure B.10 is an example of a:

    a. T1-weighted image ☐
    b. T2-weighted image ☐
    c. Spin (proton) density-weighted image ☐
    d. T2*-weighted image ☐
    e. All of the above ☐

147. On Figure B.10 arrow A is pointing to the:

    a. Oropharynx ☐
    b. Nasopharynx ☐
    c. Anterior arch of C1 ☐
    d. Dens (odontoid) ☐

148. On Figure B.10 arrow B is pointing to the:

> **a.** Oropharynx ☐
> **b.** Nasopharynx ☐
> **c.** Anterior arch of C1 ☐
> **d.** Dens (odontoid) ☐

149. On Figure B.10 arrow C is pointing to the:

> **a.** Oropharynx ☐
> **b.** Nasopharynx ☐
> **c.** Anterior arch of C1 ☐
> **d.** Dens (odontoid) ☐

150. On Figure B.10 arrow D is pointing to:

> **a.** CSF in the subarachnoid space ☐
> **b.** The cervical disk ☐
> **c.** The spinal cord ☐
> **d.** The meninges ☐

151. On Figure B.10 arrow E is pointing to the:

> **a.** Oropharynx ☐
> **b.** Nasopharynx ☐
> **c.** Trachea ☐
> **d.** Esophagus ☐

152. On Figure B.10 arrow F is pointing to the:

> **a.** Vertebral body ☐
> **b.** Spinal cord ☐
> **c.** Intervertebral disk ☐
> **d.** Spinal canal ☐

153. On Figure B.10 arrow G is pointing to the:

> **a.** Vertebral body ☐
> **b.** Spinal cord ☐
> **c.** Intervertebral disk ☐
> **d.** Spinal canal ☐

154. On Figure B.10 the vertebral bodies of the cervical spine can be visualized because:

    a. Bone is radiolucent and therefore appears dark on all MR images   ☐

    b. Bone is dense and attenuates the RF pulse, and therefore appears bright on all MR images   ☐

    c. The hydrogen in cortical bone is too tightly bound to be "excited" by the MR imaging process; therefore, cortical bone appears dark on MR images and "outlines" the vertebral body   ☐

    d. Bone marrow contains fat and water, and therefore appears bright depending upon the scan parameters used to create the image (surrounded by the "outlining of cortical bone")   ☐

    e. c and d   ☐

155. On Figure B.10 there is a "slight" cervical disk herniation (bulge) at the level of:

    a. C1/C2   ☐

    b. C2/C3   ☐

    c. C5/C6   ☐

    d. C7/T1   ☐

156. 3D gradient echo axial views can be used in cervical spine imaging to provide:

    a. Thin contiguous sections of the spine   ☐

    b. The ability to reformat into any other imaging plane, retrospectively   ☐

    c. The ability to get either T1, spin density, or T2* information by changing image acquisition parameters (TR, TE, and flip angle)   ☐

    d. All of the above   ☐

    e. a and b only   ☐

157. In complete spine imaging, to rule out metastatic lesions of the spinal cord, contrast enhancement can be used with T1-weighted images because:

    a. Normal cord enhances and metastatic lesions do not   ☐

    b. Metastatic lesions (within the cord) enhance and normal cord does not   ☐

    c. Scar enhances and disk does not   ☐

    d. CSF is bright and cord is dark   ☐

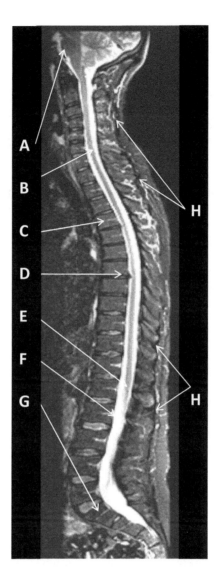

Figure B.11

158. Figure B.11 was acquired with a 48-cm rectangular FOV, 4-mm slice thickness, and a 512 × 512 imaging matrix. A small FOV image that would bear the same spatial resolution is:

    a. 24-cm FOV, 4-mm slice thickness, and a 256 × 256 matrix   ☐
    b. 48-cm FOV, 4-mm slice thickness, and a 256 × 256 matrix (without rectangular FOV)   ☐
    c. 24-cm rectangular FOV, 2-mm slice thickness, and a 256 × 256 matrix   ☐
    d. 12-cm FOV, 8-mm slice thickness, and a 512 × 512 matrix   ☐

159. Judging from the signal-to-noise ratio (SNR) on Figure B.11, the coil or coils that were most likely used to acquire this image are:

> **a.** A 5-inch surface coil ☐
> **b.** A Helmholtz coil pair ☐
> **c.** The body coil ☐
> **d.** Phased array coils ☐

160. On Figure B.11 the low signal intensity area (arrows H) that runs superior and inferior but posterior to the spinous processes represents:

> **a.** The cruciate ligament ☐
> **b.** Chemical shift artifact ☐
> **c.** The spinatus tendon ☐
> **d.** Gibbs or truncation artifact ☐

161. Figure B.11 was acquired in the:

> **a.** Axial imaging plane ☐
> **b.** Sagittal imaging plane ☐
> **c.** Coronal imaging plane ☐
> **d.** Off-axis (oblique) imaging plane ☐

162. Figure B.11 is an example of a:

> **a.** T1-weighted image (whereby fluid is dark and fat is bright) ☐
> **b.** T2-weighted image (whereby fluid is bright and fat is darker) ☐
> **c.** Spin (proton) density-weighted image (whereby both fat and fluid are bright) ☐
> **d.** FLAIR image [whereby the signal from fluid is "attenuated" or "suppressed" (dark) and the signal from fat is brighter] ☐

163. On Figure B.11 arrow A is pointing to the:

> **a.** Pituitary gland ☐
> **b.** Internal auditory canals ☐
> **c.** Pons ☐
> **d.** Cervical spinal cord ☐

164. On Figure B.11 arrow B is pointing to the:

a. Oropharynx ☐
b. Nasopharynx ☐
c. Pons ☐
d. Cervical spinal cord ☐

165. On Figure B.11 arrow C is pointing to:

a. C3 (the third cervical vertebral body) ☐
b. T3 (the third thoracic vertebral body) ☐
c. L3 (the third lumbar vertebral body) ☐
d. S3 (the third sacral vertebral body) ☐

166. On Figure B.11 arrow D is pointing to the:

a. Intervertebral disk ☐
b. Vertebral body ☐
c. Spinal cord ☐
d. Cauda equina ☐

167. On Figure B.11 arrow E is pointing to the:

a. Cervical spinal cord ☐
b. Conus medularis ☐
c. Cauda equina ☐
d. Esophagus ☐

168. On Figure B.11 arrow F is pointing to the:

a. Cervical spinal cord ☐
b. Conus medularis ☐
c. Cauda equina ☐
d. Esophagus ☐

169. On Figure B.11 arrow G is pointing to the:

a. Lumbar vertebral body ☐
b. Spinal cord ☐
c. Intervertebral disk ☐
d. Spinal canal ☐
e. Sacrum ☐

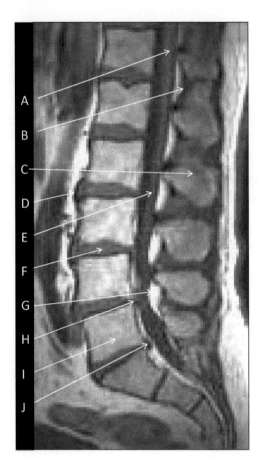

Figure B.12

170. Figure B.12 was acquired in the:

    a. Axial imaging plane ☐
    b. Sagittal imaging plane ☐
    c. Coronal imaging plane ☐
    d. Off-axis (oblique) imaging plane ☐

171. Figure B.12 is an example of a:

    a. T1-weighted image ☐
    b. T2-weighted image ☐
    c. Spin (proton) -weighted image ☐
    d. T2*-weighted image ☐
    e. All of the above ☐

172. Figure B.12 could have been acquired with a spin echo (or fast spin echo) acquisition with:

a. Short TR and short TE ☐
b. Long TR and short TE ☐
c. Short TR and long TE ☐
d. Long TR and long TE ☐

173. On Figure B.12 arrow A is pointing to:

a. Cervical spinal cord ☐
b. Conus medularis ☐
c. Cauda equina ☐
d. Posterior longitudinal ligament ☐
e. Anterior longitudinal ligament ☐

174. On Figure B.12 arrow B is pointing to the:

a. Ligamentum flavum ☐
b. Conus medularis ☐
c. Cauda equina ☐
d. Posterior longitudinal ligament ☐

175. On Figure B.12 arrow C is pointing to the:

a. Intervertebral disk ☐
b. Spinous process ☐
c. Transverse process ☐
d. Vertebral body ☐
e. Pedicle ☐

176. On Figure B.12 arrow D is pointing to the:

a. Ligamentum flavum ☐
b. Conus medularis ☐
c. Cauda equina ☐
d. Posterior longitudinal ligament ☐
e. Anterior longitudinal ligament ☐

177. On Figure B.12 arrow E is pointing to the:

    a. Ligamentum flavum ☐
    b. Conus medularis ☐
    c. Cauda equina ☐
    d. Posterior longitudinal ligament ☐
    e. Anterior longitudinal ligament ☐

178. On Figure B.12 arrow F is pointing to the:

    a. L3/L4 intervertebral disk ☐
    b. L4/L5 intervertebral disk ☐
    c. Cauda equina ☐
    d. L4 vertebral body ☐
    e. L5 vertebral body ☐

179. On Figure B.12 arrow G is pointing to:

    a. Intervertebral disk ☐
    b. Vertebral body ☐
    c. Spinal Cord ☐
    d. Epidural fat ☐
    e. Cerebrospinal fluid (CSF) ☐

180. On Figure B.12 arrow H is pointing to the:

    a. Ligamentum flavum ☐
    b. Conus medularis ☐
    c. Cauda equina ☐
    d. Posterior longitudinal ligament ☐
    e. Anterior longitudinal ligament ☐

181. On Figure B.12 arrow I is pointing to the:

    a. L3/L4 intervertebral disk ☐
    b. L4/L5 intervertebral disk ☐
    c. Cauda equina ☐
    d. L4 vertebral body ☐
    e. L5 vertebral body ☐

182. On Figure B.12 arrow J is pointing to the intervertebral disk at the level of:

    a. L2/L3 ☐
    b. L3/L4 ☐
    c. L4/L5 ☐
    d. L5/S1 ☐

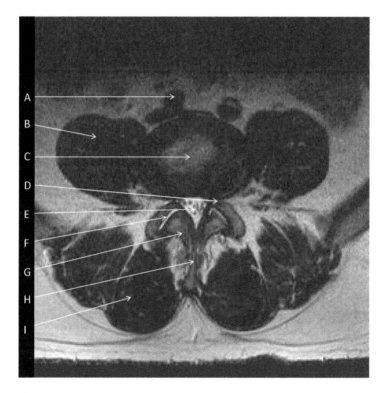

Figure B.13

183. To evaluate the intervertebral disk in the lumbar spine, imaging (Figure B.13) is generally performed in the:

    a. Axial imaging plane ☐
    b. Sagittal imaging plane ☐
    c. Coronal imaging plane ☐
    d. Off-axis (oblique) imaging plane ☐

184. Figure B.13 is an example of a:

- **a.** T1-weighted image ☐
- **b.** T2-weighted image ☐
- **c.** Spin (proton) density-weighted image ☐
- **d.** FLAIR weighted image ☐

185. Figure B.13could have been acquired with spin echo (or fast spin echo) with:

- **a.** Short TR and short TE ☐
- **b.** Long TR and short TE ☐
- **c.** Short TR and long TE ☐
- **d.** Long TR and long TE ☐

186. On Figure B.13 arrow A is pointing to the:

- **a.** Abdominal aorta ☐
- **b.** Right common iliac artery ☐
- **c.** Left common iliac artery ☐
- **d.** Inferior vena cava (IVC) ☐

187. On Figure B.13 arrow B is pointing to the:

- **a.** Right gluteal muscle ☐
- **b.** Left gluteal muscle ☐
- **c.** Right erector spinae muscle ☐
- **d.** Left erector spinae muscle ☐
- **e.** Right psoas muscle ☐
- **f.** Left psoas muscle ☐

188. On Figure B.13 arrow C is pointing to the:

- **a.** Vertebral body ☐
- **b.** Left gluteal muscle ☐
- **c.** Intervertebral disk ☐
- **d.** Pedicle ☐
- **e.** Lamina ☐

189. On Figure B.13 arrow D is pointing to the:

> **a.** Vertebral body ☐
> **b.** Left gluteal muscle ☐
> **c.** Intervertebral disk ☐
> **d.** Pedicle ☐
> **e.** Lamina ☐

190. On Figure B.13 arrow E is pointing to the:

> **a.** Spinal cord ☐
> **b.** Vertebral body ☐
> **c.** Intervertebral disk ☐
> **d.** Spinal canal (with nerve roots) ☐

191. On Figure B.13 arrow F is pointing to:

> **a.** Posterior longitudinal ligament ☐
> **b.** Facet joint ☐
> **c.** Zygapophyseal joint ☐
> **d.** b and c ☐

192. On Figure B.13 arrow G is pointing to:

> **a.** Vertebral body ☐
> **b.** Left gluteal muscle ☐
> **c.** Intervertebral disk ☐
> **d.** Pedicle ☐
> **e.** Lamina ☐

193. On Figure B.13 arrow H is pointing to the:

> **a.** Intervertebral disk ☐
> **b.** Spinous process ☐
> **c.** Transverse process ☐
> **d.** Vertebral body ☐
> **e.** Pedicle ☐

194. On Figure B.13 arrow I is pointing to the:

    a. Right gluteal muscle ☐
    b. Left gluteal muscle ☐
    c. Right erector spinae muscle ☐
    d. Left erector spinae muscle ☐
    e. Right psoas muscle ☐
    f. Left psoas muscle ☐

MRI of the thorax

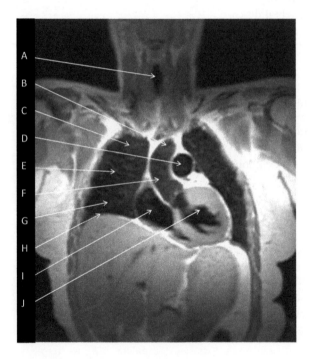

Figure B.14

195. Figure B.14 was acquired in the:

    a. Axial imaging plane ☐
    b. Sagittal imaging plane ☐
    c. Coronal imaging plane ☐
    d. Off-axis (oblique) imaging plane ☐

196. Figure B.14 is an example of a:

> **a.** T1-weighted image ☐
> **b.** T2-weighted image ☐
> **c.** Spin (proton) density-weighted image ☐
> **d.** T2*-weighted image ☐

197. On Figure B.14 arrow A is pointing to the:

> **a.** Trachea ☐
> **b.** Esophagus ☐
> **c.** Thyroid gland ☐
> **d.** Carotid artery ☐

198. On Figure B.14 arrow B is pointing to the:

> **a.** Ascending aorta ☐
> **b.** Aortic arch ☐
> **c.** Thoracic aorta ☐
> **d.** Pulmonary artery ☐

199. On Figure B.14 arrow C is pointing to the:

> **a.** Superior lobe of the right lung (apex) ☐
> **b.** Superior lobe of the left lung (apex) ☐
> **c.** Middle lobe of the right lung ☐
> **d.** Middle lobe of the left lung ☐
> **e.** Inferior lobe of the right lung (base) ☐
> **f.** Inferior lobe of the left lung (base) ☐

200. On Figure B.14 there is no signal arising from within the lung (indicated by arrows C, E, and G) because:

> **a.** There are no protons in air ☐
> **b.** There is no air in the lung during image acquisition ☐
> **c.** There are not enough mobile protons in air ☐
> **d.** Air and moving blood have the same number of protons and, therefore, both appear black ☐

201. On Figure B.14 arrow D is pointing to the:

a. Ascending aorta ☐
b. Aortic arch ☐
c. Thoracic aorta ☐
d. Pulmonary artery ☐

202. On Figure B.14 arrow E is pointing to the:

a. Superior lobe of the right lung (apex) ☐
b. Superior lobe of the left lung (apex) ☐
c. Middle lobe of the right lung ☐
d. Middle lobe of the left lung ☐
e. Inferior lobe of the right lung (base) ☐
f. Inferior lobe of the left lung (base) ☐

203. On Figure B.14 arrow F is pointing to the:

a. Ascending aorta ☐
b. Aortic arch ☐
c. Thoracic aorta ☐
d. Pulmonary artery ☐

204. On Figure B.14 arrow G is pointing to the:

a. Superior lobe of the right lung (apex) ☐
b. Superior lobe of the left lung (apex) ☐
c. Middle lobe of the right lung ☐
d. Middle lobe of the left lung ☐
e. Inferior lobe of the right lung (base) ☐
f. Inferior lobe of the left lung (base) ☐

205. On Figure B.14 arrow H is pointing to the:

a. Base of the right lung ☐
b. Apex of the right lung ☐
c. Diaphragm ☐
d. Right main pulmonary artery ☐

206. On Figure B.14 arrow I is pointing to the:

a. Right atrium ☐
b. Left atrium ☐
c. Right ventricle ☐
d. Left ventricle ☐

207. On Figure B.14 arrow J is pointing to the:

a. Right apex ☐
b. Left apex ☐
c. Right ventricle ☐
d. Left ventricle ☐

208. To minimize pulsatile flow motion artifacts, cardiac images are acquired by:

a. Taking the patient's pulse, calculating the heart rate in beats per minute, then entering these data into the imaging system ☐
b. Cardiac gating (or triggering) – attach ECG leads, monitor the cardiac cycle, and "time" the scan or "trigger" the scan from the heart beat ☐
c. Performing cardiopulmonary resuscitation ☐
d. None of the above ☐

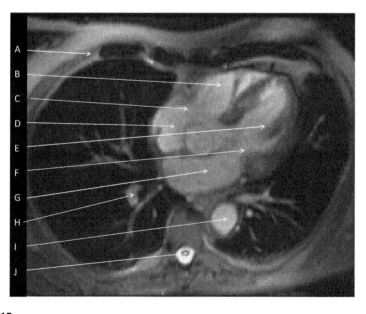

Figure B.15

209. Figure B.15 was acquired in the:

> **a.** Axial imaging plane ☐
> **b.** Sagittal imaging plane ☐
> **c.** Coronal imaging plane ☐
> **d.** Off-axis (oblique) imaging plane ☐

210. Figure B.15 is an example of a:

> **a.** Spin echo acquisition ☐
> **b.** Fast spin echo acquisition ☐
> **c.** FLAIR acquisition ☐
> **d.** Gradient echo acquisition ☐

211. On Figure B.15 arrow A is pointing to the:

> **a.** Gluteal muscles ☐
> **b.** Intercostal muscles ☐
> **c.** Spinal muscles ☐
> **d.** Pectoralis muscles ☐

212. On Figure B.15 arrow B is pointing to the:

> **a.** Right atrium ☐
> **b.** Tricuspid valve ☐
> **c.** Right ventricle ☐
> **d.** Left atrium ☐
> **e.** Left ventricle ☐
> **f.** Bicuspid valve ☐

213. On Figure B.15 arrow C is pointing to the:

> **a.** Right atrium ☐
> **b.** Tricuspid valve ☐
> **c.** Right ventricle ☐
> **d.** Left atrium ☐
> **e.** Left ventricle ☐
> **f.** Bicuspid valve ☐

214. On Figure B.15 arrow D is pointing to the:

- **a.** Right atrium ☐
- **b.** Tricuspid valve ☐
- **c.** Right ventricle ☐
- **d.** Left atrium ☐
- **e.** Left ventricle ☐
- **f.** Bicuspid valve ☐

215. On Figure B.15 arrow E is pointing to the:

- **a.** Right atrium ☐
- **b.** Tricuspid valve ☐
- **c.** Right ventricle ☐
- **d.** Left atrium ☐
- **e.** Left ventricle ☐
- **f.** Bicuspid valve ☐

216. On Figure B.15 arrow F is pointing to the:

- **a.** Right atrium ☐
- **b.** Tricuspid valve ☐
- **c.** Right ventricle ☐
- **d.** Left atrium ☐
- **e.** Left ventricle ☐
- **f.** Bicuspid valve ☐

217. On Figure B.15 arrow G is pointing to the:

- **a.** Right atrium ☐
- **b.** Tricuspid valve ☐
- **c.** Right ventricle ☐
- **d.** Left atrium ☐
- **e.** Left ventricle ☐
- **f.** Bicuspid valve ☐

218. On Figure B.15 arrow H is pointing to the:

- **a.** Thoracic aorta ☐
- **b.** Pulmonary artery ☐
- **c.** Spinal canal ☐
- **d.** Left atrium ☐

219. On Figure B.15 arrow I is pointing to the:

    a. Thoracic aorta ☐
    b. Pulmonary artery ☐
    c. Spinal canal ☐
    d. Left atrium ☐

220. On Figure B.15 arrow J is pointing to the:

    a. Thoracic aorta ☐
    b. Pulmonary artery ☐
    c. Spinal canal ☐
    d. Left atrium ☐

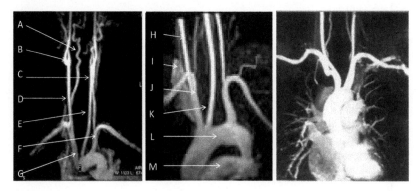

Figure B.16

221. On Figure B.16 arrow A is pointing to the:

    a. Right vertebral artery ☐
    b. Left vertebral artery ☐
    c. Right common carotid artery ☐
    d. Left common carotid artery ☐
    e. Right carotid bifurcation ☐

222. On Figure B.16 arrow B is pointing to the:

    a. Right vertebral artery ☐
    b. Left vertebral artery ☐
    c. Right common carotid artery ☐
    d. Left common carotid artery ☐
    e. Right carotid bifurcation ☐

223. On Figure B.16 arrow C is pointing to the:

a. Right vertebral artery ☐
b. Left vertebral artery ☐
c. Right common carotid artery ☐
d. Left common carotid artery ☐
e. Right carotid bifurcation ☐

224. On Figure B.16 arrow D is pointing to the:

a. Right vertebral artery ☐
b. Left vertebral artery ☐
c. Right common carotid artery ☐
d. Left common carotid artery ☐
e. Right carotid bifurcation ☐

225. On Figure B.16 arrow E is pointing to the:

a. Right vertebral artery ☐
b. Left vertebral artery ☐
c. Right common carotid artery ☐
d. Left common carotid artery ☐
e. Right carotid bifurcation ☐

226. On Figure B.16 arrow F is pointing to the:

a. Right subclavian artery ☐
b. Left subclavian artery ☐
c. Right inominate carotid artery ☐
d. Left inominate carotid artery ☐

227. On Figure B.16 arrow G is pointing to the:

a. Right subclavian artery ☐
b. Left subclavian artery ☐
c. Inominate artery ☐
d. Left inominate carotid artery ☐

228. On Figure B.16 arrow H is pointing to the:

    a. Superior vena cava ☐
    b. Right vertebral artery ☐
    c. Right common carotid artery ☐
    d. Left common carotid artery ☐

229. On Figure B.16 arrow I is pointing to the:

    a. Superior vena cava ☐
    b. Inferior vena cava ☐
    c. Pulmonary artery ☐
    d. Aortic arch ☐

230. On Figure B.16 arrow J is pointing to the:

    a. Brachiocephalic artery ☐
    b. Innominate artery ☐
    c. Right vertebral artery ☐
    d. a and b ☐

231. On Figure B.16 arrow K is pointing to the:

    a. Superior vena cava ☐
    b. Right vertebral artery ☐
    c. Right common carotid artery ☐
    d. Left common carotid artery ☐

232. On Figure B.16 arrow L is pointing to the:

    a. Superior vena cava ☐
    b. Inferior vena cava ☐
    c. Pulmonary artery ☐
    d. Aortic arch ☐

233. On Figure B.16 arrow M is pointing to the:

    a. Superior vena cava ☐
    b. Inferior vena cava ☐
    c. Pulmonary artery ☐
    d. Aortic arch ☐

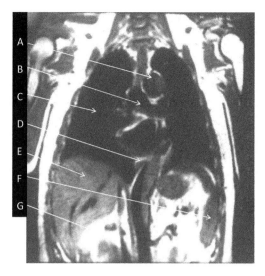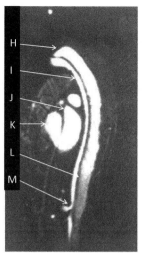

Figure B.17

234. On Figure B.17 arrow A is pointing to the:

    a. Ascending aorta ☐
    b. Aortic arch ☐
    c. Descending aorta ☐
    d. Abdominal aorta ☐
    e. Superior mesenteric artery ☐

235. The optimal view (or views) for the evaluation of the aortic arch include:
    1. Sagittal
    2. Axial
    3. Coronal
    4. Oblique

    a. 1 only ☐
    b. 2 only ☐
    c. 1 and 3 only ☐
    d. 1 and 4 only ☐

236. On Figure B.17 arrow B is pointing to the:

    a. Ascending aorta ☐
    b. Aortic arch ☐
    c. Descending aorta ☐
    d. Abdominal aorta ☐
    e. Pulmonary artery ☐

237. On Figure B.17 arrow C is pointing to the:

 a. Right atrium ☐
 b. Left atrium ☐
 c. Right ventricle ☐
 d. Left ventricle ☐
 e. Right lung ☐
 f. Left lung ☐

238. On Figure B.17 arrow D is pointing to the:

 a. Ascending aorta ☐
 b. Aortic arch ☐
 c. Descending aorta ☐
 d. Abdominal aorta ☐
 e. Superior mesenteric artery ☐

239. On Figure B.17 arrow E is pointing to the:

 a. Liver ☐
 b. Spleen ☐
 c. Kidney ☐
 d. Retroperitoneal fat ☐

240. On Figure B.17 arrow F is pointing to the:

 a. Liver ☐
 b. Spleen ☐
 c. Kidney ☐
 d. Retroperitoneal fat ☐

241. On Figure B.17 arrow G is pointing to the:

 a. Liver ☐
 b. Spleen ☐
 c. Kidney ☐
 d. Retroperitoneal fat ☐

242. On Figure B.17 arrow H is pointing to the:

a. Ascending aorta ☐
b. Aortic arch ☐
c. Descending aorta ☐
d. Abdominal aorta ☐
e. Superior mesenteric artery ☐

243. On Figure B.17 arrow I is pointing to the:

a. Ascending aorta ☐
b. Aortic arch ☐
c. Descending aorta ☐
d. Abdominal aorta ☐
e. Superior mesenteric artery ☐

244. On Figure B.17 arrow **J** is pointing to the most posterior chamber of the heart, which is the:

a. Right atrium ☐
b. Left atrium ☐
c. Right ventricle ☐
d. Left ventricle ☐
e. Right lung ☐
f. Left lung ☐

245. On Figure B.17 arrow K is pointing to the most anterior chamber of the heart, which is the:

a. Right atrium ☐
b. Left atrium ☐
c. Right ventricle ☐
d. Left ventricle ☐
e. Right lung ☐
f. Left lung ☐

246. On Figure B.17 arrow L is pointing to the:

a. Ascending aorta ☐
b. Aortic arch ☐
c. Descending aorta ☐
d. Abdominal aorta ☐
e. Superior mesenteric artery ☐

247. On Figure B.17 arrow M is pointing to the:

a. Ascending aorta ☐
b. Aortic arch ☐
c. Descending aorta ☐
d. Abdominal aorta ☐
e. Superior mesenteric artery ☐

Cardiac Views

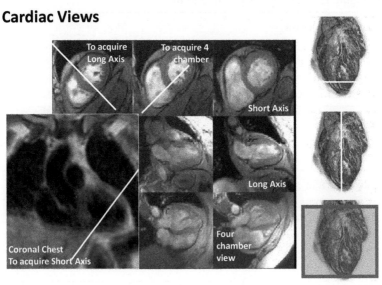

Cardiac Energetics, NHLBI

Figure B.18

248. On Figure B.18 the SHORT AXIS views of the heart resemble images that are:

a. Axial to the plane of the heart muscle ☐
b. Sagittal to the plane of the heart muscle ☐
c. Coronal to the plane of the heart muscle ☐
d. Axial to the plane of the aorta ☐

249. On Figure B.18 the LONG AXIS views of the heart resemble images that are:

a. Axial to the plane of the heart muscle ☐
b. Sagittal to the plane of the heart muscle ☐
c. Coronal to the plane of the heart muscle ☐
d. Axial to the plane of the aorta ☐

250. On Figure B.18 the FOUR CHAMBER views of the heart resemble images that are:

    a. Axial to the plane of the heart muscle ☐
    b. Sagittal to the plane of the heart muscle ☐
    c. Coronal to the plane of the heart muscle ☐
    d. Axial to the plane of the aorta ☐

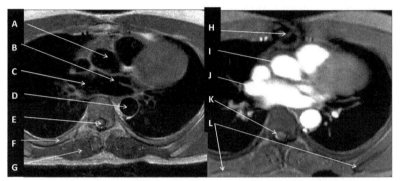

Gated Spin Echo
TR = 1 R-R (~940 msec) TE = 14

Cine Phase Contrast
TR 5.6, TE 3.6 flip angle 30°

Figure B.19

251. On Figure B.19 arrow A is pointing to the:

    a. Ascending aorta ☐
    b. Right pulmonary artery ☐
    c. Left pulmonary artery ☐
    d. Descending thoracic aorta ☐

252. On Figure B.19 arrow B is pointing to the:

    a. Ascending aorta ☐
    b. Right pulmonary artery ☐
    c. Left pulmonary artery ☐
    d. Descending thoracic aorta ☐

253. On Figure B.19 arrow C is pointing to the:

    a. Ascending aorta ☐
    b. Right pulmonary artery ☐
    c. Left pulmonary artery ☐
    d. Descending thoracic aorta ☐

254. On Figure B.19 arrow D is pointing to the:

a. Ascending aorta ☐
b. Right pulmonary artery ☐
c. Left pulmonary artery ☐
d. Descending thoracic aorta ☐

255. On Figure B.19 arrow E is pointing to the:

a. Spinal muscles ☐
b. Spinal canal ☐
c. Vertebral body ☐
d. Rib ☐

256. On Figure B.19 arrow F is pointing to the:

a. Spinal muscles ☐
b. Spinal canal ☐
c. Vertebral body ☐
d. Rib ☐

257. On Figure B.19 arrow G is pointing to the:

a. Spinal muscles ☐
b. Spinal canal ☐
c. Vertebral body ☐
d. Rib ☐

258. On Figure B.19 (the gradient echo image – right) arrow H is pointing to the:

a. Susceptibility artifact ☐
b. Bright signal from flowing blood – ascending aorta ☐
c. Bright signal from flowing blood – pulmonary artery ☐
d. Bright signal from flowing CSF in the spinal canal ☐
e. Chemical shift artifact ☐

259. On Figure B.19 (the gradient echo image – right) arrow I is pointing to the:

a. Susceptibility artifact ☐
b. Bright signal from flowing blood – ascending aorta ☐
c. Bright signal from flowing blood – pulmonary artery ☐
d. Bright signal from flowing CSF in the spinal canal ☐
e. Chemical shift artifact ☐

260. On Figure B.19 (the gradient echo image – right) arrow J is pointing to the:

a. Susceptibility artifact ☐
b. Bright signal from flowing blood – ascending aorta ☐
c. Bright signal from flowing blood – pulmonary artery ☐
d. Bright signal from flowing CSF in the spinal canal ☐
e. Chemical shift artifact ☐

261. On Figure B.19 (the gradient echo image – right) arrow K is pointing to the:

a. Susceptibility artifact ☐
b. Bright signal from flowing blood – ascending aorta ☐
c. Bright signal from flowing blood – pulmonary artery ☐
d. Bright signal from flowing CSF in the spinal canal ☐
e. Chemical shift artifact ☐

262. On Figure B.19 (the gradient echo image – right) arrow L is pointing to the:

a. Susceptibility artifact ☐
b. Bright signal from flowing blood – ascending aorta ☐
c. Bright signal from flowing blood – pulmonary artery ☐
d. Bright signal from flowing CSF in the spinal canal ☐
e. Chemical shift artifact ☐

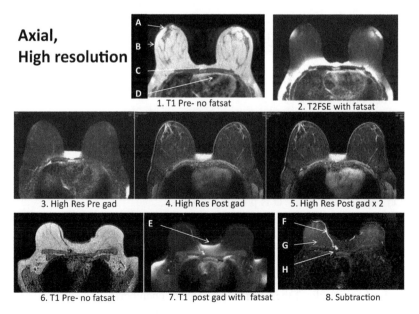

Axial,
High resolution

1. T1 Pre- no fatsat
2. T2FSE with fatsat
3. High Res Pre gad
4. High Res Post gad
5. High Res Post gad x 2
6. T1 Pre- no fatsat
7. T1 post gad with fatsat
8. Subtraction

Figure B.20

263. On Figure B.20 arrow A is pointing to the:

a. Nipple ☐
b. Fatty tissue of the breast ☐
c. Pectoralis muscle ☐
d. Shading from fat suppression ☐
e. Neovascularity ☐
f. Enhancing breast lesion ☐

264. The images in Figure B.20 have been acquired with:

a. Sagittal high-resolution imaging ☐
b. Axial high-resolution imaging ☐
c. Coronal high-resolution imaging ☐
d. Oblique high-resolution imaging ☐

265. On Figure B.20 arrow B is pointing to the:

a. Nipple ☐
b. Fatty tissue of the breast ☐
c. Pectoralis muscle ☐
d. Shading from fat suppression ☐
e. Neovascularity ☐
f. Enhancing breast lesion ☐

266. On Figure B.20 arrow C is pointing to the:

a. Nipple ☐
b. Fatty tissue of the breast ☐
c. Pectoralis muscle ☐
d. Ducts and lobules ☐
e. Neovascularity ☐
f. Enhancing breast lesion ☐

267. On Figure B.20 arrow D is pointing to the:

a. Nipple ☐
b. Fatty tissue of the breast ☐
c. Pectoralis muscle ☐
d. Shading from fat suppression ☐
e. Right ventricle of the heart (most anterior chamber) ☐
f. Left atrium of the heart (most anterior chamber) ☐

268. On Figure B.20 arrow E is pointing to the:

   a. Nipple ☐
   b. Fatty tissue of the breast ☐
   c. Pectoralis muscle ☐
   d. Shading from fat suppression ☐
   e. Neovascularity ☐
   f. Enhancing breast lesion ☐

269. On Figure B.20 arrow F is pointing to the:

   a. Fatty tissue of the breast ☐
   b. Pectoralis muscle ☐
   c. Shading from fat suppression ☐
   d. Neovascularity ☐
   e. Enhancing breast lesion ☐

270. On Figure B.20 arrow G is pointing to the:

   a. Fatty tissue of the breast ☐
   b. Pectoralis muscle ☐
   c. Shading from fat suppression ☐
   d. Neovascularity ☐
   e. Enhancing breast lesion ☐

271. On Figure B.20 arrow H is pointing to the:

   a. Fatty issue of the breast ☐
   b. Pectoralis muscles ☐
   c. Shading from fat suppression ☐
   d. Neovascularity ☐
   e. Enhancing breast lesion ☐

272. On Figure B.20 the following images were acquired WITH fat suppression:

   a. 1 and 2 ☐
   b. 3, 4 and 5 ☐
   c. 6, 7 and 8 ☐
   d. 2, 3, 4, 5, 7, and 8 ☐
   e. 1 and 6 ☐

273. On Figure B.20 the following images were acquired WITHOUT fat suppression:

a. 1 and 2 ☐
b. 3, 4, and 5 ☐
c. 6, 7, and 8 ☐
d. 2, 3, 4, 5, 7, and 8 ☐
e. 1 and 6 ☐

274. On Figure B.21 arrow A is pointing to the:

a. Nipple ☐
b. Fatty tissue of the breast ☐
c. Pectoralis muscle ☐
d. Ducts and lobules ☐
e. Neovascularity ☐
f. Enhancing breast lesion ☐

Sagittal Breast Protocol

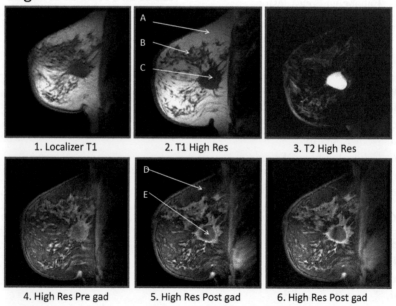

1. Localizer T1   2. T1 High Res   3. T2 High Res

4. High Res Pre gad   5. High Res Post gad   6. High Res Post gad

Figure B.21

275. The images in Figure B.21 have been acquired with:

    a. Sagittal high-resolution imaging ☐
    b. Axial high-resolution imaging ☐
    c. Coronal high-resolution imaging ☐
    d. Oblique high-resolution imaging ☐

276. On Figure B.21 arrow B is pointing to the:

    a. Nipple ☐
    b. Fatty tissue of the breast ☐
    c. Pectoralis muscle ☐
    d. Ducts and lobules ☐
    e. Neovascularity ☐
    f. Enhancing breast lesion ☐

277. On Figure B.21 arrow D is pointing to the:

    a. Nipple ☐
    b. Fatty tissue of the breast ☐
    c. Pectoralis muscle ☐
    d. Ducts and lobules ☐
    e. Neovascularity ☐
    f. Enhancing breast lesion ☐

278. On Figure B.21 arrow E is pointing to the:

    a. Nipple ☐
    b. Fatty tissue of the breast ☐
    c. Pectoralis muscle ☐
    d. Ducts and lobules ☐
    e. Neovascularity ☐
    f. Enhancing breast lesion ☐

279. On Figure B.21 the following images were acquired WITH fat suppression:

    a. 1, 2, and 3   ☐
    b. 4, 5, and 6   ☐
    c. 1 and 2   ☐
    d. 3, 4, 5, and 6   ☐

280. On Figure B.21 the following images were acquired WITHOUT fat suppression:

    a. 1, 2, and 3   ☐
    b. 4, 5, and 6   ☐
    c. 1 and 2   ☐
    d. 3, 4, 5, and 6   ☐

Extra Capsular Rupture

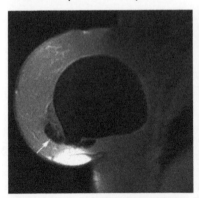 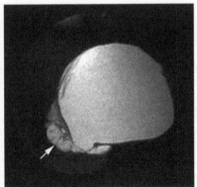

Silicone suppression   Fat & Water Suppression

Figure B.22

281. Figure B.22 shows high-resolution sagittal images of the breast in a patient with silicone implants with:

- **a.** Fat suppression ☐
- **b.** Water suppression ☐
- **c.** Silicone suppression ☐
- **d.** Silicone, water, and fat suppression ☐

282. Review Figure B.22 (right). Images for the evaluation of silicone implants, whereby the silicone is to appear bright, should be acquired with the application of:
1. Fat suppression
2. Water suppression
3. Silicone suppression

- **a.** 1 only ☐
- **b.** 1 and 2 only ☐
- **c.** 3 only ☐
- **d.** 1 and 3 only ☐
- **e.** 1, 2, and 3 ☐

283. Review Figure B.22 (left). Images for the evaluation of silicone implants, whereby the silicone is to appear dark, should be acquired with the application of:
1. Fat suppression
2. Water suppression
3. Silicone suppression

- **a.** 1 only ☐
- **b.** 1 and 2 only ☐
- **c.** 3 only ☐
- **d.** 1 and 3 only ☐
- **e.** 1, 2, and 3 ☐

MRI of the abdomen and pelvis

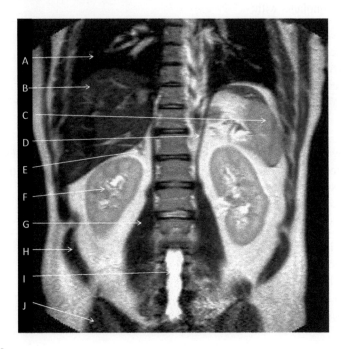

Figure B.23

284. Figure B.23 was acquired in the:

a. Axial imaging plane	☐
b. Sagittal imaging plane	☐
c. Coronal imaging plane	☐
d. Off-axis (oblique) imaging plane	☐

285. Figure B.23 is an example of a:

a. T1-weighted image	☐
b. T2-weighted image	☐
c. Spin (proton) density-weighted image	☐
d. FLAIR image	☐

286. On Figure B.23 arrow A is pointing to the:

 a. Left kidney ☐
 b. Spleen ☐
 c. Liver ☐
 d. Stomach ☐
 e. Right lung ☐

287. Figure B.23 was acquired with:

 a. Short TR, short TE with fat suppression ☐
 b. Short TR, short TE with water suppression ☐
 c. Long TR, long TE with fat suppression ☐
 d. Long TR, long TE with no suppression ☐

288. On Figure B.23 arrow B is pointing to the:

 a. Left kidney ☐
 b. Spleen ☐
 c. Liver ☐
 d. Stomach ☐
 e. Right lung ☐

289. On Figure B.23 arrow C is pointing to the:

 a. Left kidney ☐
 b. Spleen ☐
 c. Liver ☐
 d. Stomach ☐
 e. Right lung ☐

290. On Figure B.23 arrow D is pointing to the:

 a. Right adrenal gland ☐
 b. Left adrenal gland ☐
 c. Liver ☐
 d. Stomach ☐
 e. Crux (cruz) of the diaphragm ☐

291. On Figure B.23 arrow E is pointing to the:

a. Right adrenal gland ☐
b. Left adrenal gland ☐
c. Liver ☐
d. Stomach ☐
e. Crux (cruz) of the diaphragm ☐

292. On Figure B.23 arrow F is pointing to the:

a. Kidney ☐
b. Spleen ☐
c. Liver ☐
d. Stomach ☐
e. Right lung ☐

293. On Figure B.23 arrow G is pointing to the:

a. Psoas muscle ☐
b. Rectus abdominus muscle ☐
c. Oblique abdominal muscle ☐
d. Gluteal muscle ☐

294. On Figure B.23 arrow H is pointing to the:

a. Psoas muscle ☐
b. Rectus abdominus muscle ☐
c. Oblique abdominal muscle ☐
d. Gluteal muscle ☐

295. On Figure B.23 the high signal arising within the abdomen, indicated by arrow I, represents:

a. Peritonitis ☐
b. CSF in the spinal canal ☐
c. Abdominal ascites ☐
d. Retroperitoneal fat ☐

296. On Figure B.23 arrow J is pointing to the:

a. Psoas muscle ☐
b. Rectus abdominus muscle ☐
c. Oblique abdominal muscle ☐
d. Gluteal muscle ☐

297. The FDA-approved (iron oxide) oral contrast agent used for MRI makes bowel appear:

    a. Bright on T1-/bright on T2-weighted images ☐
    b. Dark on T1-/dark on T2-weighted images ☐
    c. Bright on T1-/dark on T2-weighted images ☐
    d. Dark on T1-/bright on T2-weighted images ☐

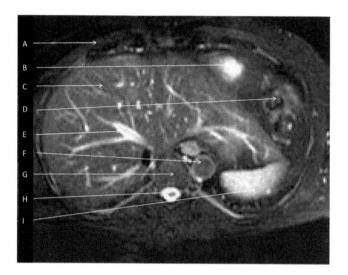

Figure B.24

298. Figure B.24 was acquired in the:

    a. Axial imaging plane ☐
    b. Sagittal imaging plane ☐
    c. Coronal imaging plane ☐
    d. Off-axis (oblique) imaging plane ☐

299. Figure B.24 is a gradient echo image acquired with:

    a. Fat suppression ☐
    b. Water suppression ☐
    c. No suppression techniques ☐
    d. Silicone suppression ☐

300. On Figure B.24 arrow A is pointing to the:

> **a.** Abdominal muscles ☐
> **b.** Stomach ☐
> **c.** Bowel ☐
> **d.** Liver ☐
> **e.** Spleen ☐

301. On Figure B.24 arrow B is pointing to the:

> **a.** Abdominal muscles ☐
> **b.** Stomach ☐
> **c.** Bowel ☐
> **d.** Liver ☐
> **e.** Spleen ☐

302. On Figure B.24 arrow C is pointing to the:

> **a.** Abdominal muscles ☐
> **b.** Stomach ☐
> **c.** Bowel ☐
> **d.** Liver ☐
> **e.** Spleen ☐

303. On Figure B.24 arrow D is pointing to the:

> **a.** Abdominal muscles ☐
> **b.** Stomach ☐
> **c.** Bowel ☐
> **d.** Liver ☐
> **e.** Spleen ☐

304. On Figure B.24 arrow E is pointing to the:

> **a.** Portal vein ☐
> **b.** Aorta ☐
> **c.** Vertebral body ☐
> **d.** Spinal cord ☐
> **e.** Hepatic artery ☐

305. On Figure B.24 arrow F is pointing to the:

a. Portal vein ☐
b. Aorta ☐
c. Vertebral body ☐
d. Spinal cord ☐
e. Hepatic artery ☐

306. On Figure B.24 arrow G is pointing to the:

a. Portal vein ☐
b. Aorta ☐
c. Vertebral body ☐
d. Spinal cord ☐
e. Hepatic artery ☐

307. On Figure B.24 arrow H is pointing to the:

a. Portal vein ☐
b. Aorta ☐
c. Vertebral body ☐
d. Spinal cord ☐
e. Hepatic artery ☐

308. On Figure B.24 arrow I is pointing to the:

a. Abdominal muscles ☐
b. Stomach ☐
c. Bowel ☐
d. Liver ☐
e. Spleen ☐

309. Due to its size and orientation within the body, the entire pancreas can possibly be visualized on one imaging section if it is acquired:

a. Coronally with thin imaging sections ☐
b. Sagittally with thin imaging sections ☐
c. Axially with thin imaging sections ☐
d. Obliquely with thick imaging sections ☐

310. On T2-weighted MR images, hemangiomas of the liver appear:

    a. Hyperintense to normal liver ☐
    b. Hypointense to normal liver ☐
    c. Isointense to normal liver ☐
    d. Only with contrast enhancement ☐

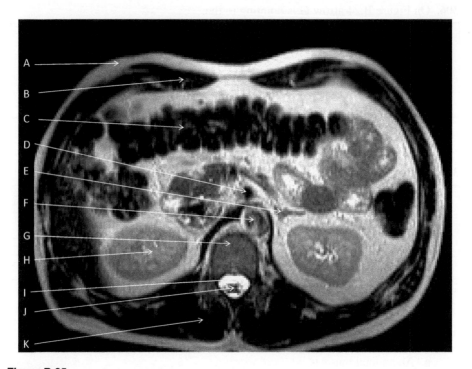

Figure B.25

311. On Figure B.25 arrow A is pointing to the:

    a. Subcutaneous fat ☐
    b. Abdominal muscles ☐
    c. Transverse colon ☐
    d. Superior mesenteric artery ☐
    e. Abdominal aorta ☐

312. On Figure B.25 arrow B is pointing to the:

a. Subcutaneous fat ☐
b. Abdominal muscles ☐
c. Transverse colon ☐
d. Superior mesenteric artery ☐
e. Abdominal aorta ☐

313. On Figure B.25 arrow C is pointing to the:

a. Stomach ☐
b. Abdominal muscles ☐
c. Transverse colon ☐
d. Superior mesenteric artery ☐
e. Abdominal aorta ☐

314. On Figure B.25 arrow D is pointing to the:

a. Superior mesenteric artery ☐
b. Abdominal aorta ☐
c. Vertebral body ☐
d. Spinal cord ☐
e. Erector spinae muscles ☐

315. On Figure B.25 arrow E is pointing to the:

a. Pancreas ☐
b. Liver ☐
c. Spleen ☐
d. Adrenal gland ☐
e. Kidney ☐

316. On Figure B.25 arrow F is pointing to the:

a. Superior mesenteric artery ☐
b. Abdominal aorta ☐
c. Vertebral body ☐
d. Spinal cord ☐
e. Erector spinae muscles ☐

317. On Figure B.25 arrow G is pointing to the:

   a. Superior mesenteric artery   ☐
   b. Abdominal aorta   ☐
   c. Vertebral body   ☐
   d. Spinal cord   ☐

318. On Figure B.25 arrow H is pointing to the:

   a. Right kidney   ☐
   b. Left kidney   ☐
   c. Right adrenal gland   ☐
   d. Right adrenal gland   ☐
   e. Pancreas   ☐

319. On Figure B.25 arrow I is pointing to the:

   a. Vertebral body   ☐
   b. Spinal cord   ☐
   c. Spinal canal   ☐
   d. Erector spinae muscles   ☐

320. On Figure B.25 arrow J is pointing to the:

   a. Vertebral body   ☐
   b. Spinal cord   ☐
   c. Spinal canal   ☐
   d. Erector spinae muscles   ☐

321. On Figure B.25 arrow K is pointing to the:

   a. Vertebral body   ☐
   b. Spinal cord   ☐
   c. Spinal canal   ☐
   d. Erector spinae muscles   ☐

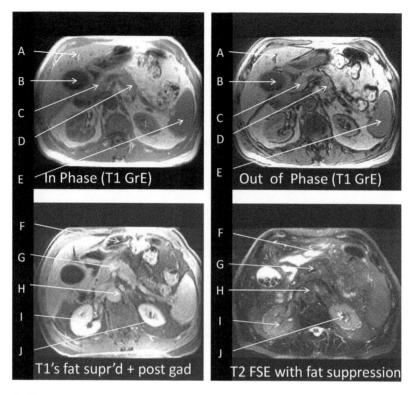

Figure B.26

322. On Figure B.26 arrow A is pointing to the:

 a. Liver ☐
 b. Spleen ☐
 c. Gallbladder ☐
 d. Head of the pancreas ☐
 e. Body of the pancreas ☐
 f. Tail of the pancreas ☐

323. On Figure B.26 arrow B is pointing to the:

 a. Liver ☐
 b. Spleen ☐
 c. Gallbladder ☐
 d. Head of the pancreas ☐
 e. Body of the pancreas ☐
 f. Tail of the pancreas ☐

324. On Figure B.26 arrow C is pointing to the:

   a. Liver ☐
   b. Spleen ☐
   c. Gallbladder ☐
   d. Head of the pancreas ☐
   e. Body of the pancreas ☐
   f. Tail of the pancreas ☐

325. On Figure B.26 arrow D is pointing to the:

   a. Liver ☐
   b. Spleen ☐
   c. Gallbladder ☐
   d. Head of the pancreas ☐
   e. Body of the pancreas ☐
   f. Tail of the pancreas ☐

326. On Figure B.26 arrow E is pointing to the:

   a. Liver ☐
   b. Spleen ☐
   c. Gallbladder ☐
   d. Head of the pancreas ☐
   e. Body of the pancreas ☐
   f. Tail of the pancreas ☐

327. On Figure B.26 arrow F is pointing to the:

   a. Liver ☐
   b. Spleen ☐
   c. Stomach ☐
   d. Colon ☐
   e. Gallbladder ☐

328. On Figure B.26 arrow G is pointing to the:

> **a.** Gallbladder ☐
> **b.** Head of the pancreas ☐
> **c.** Body of the pancreas ☐
> **d.** Tail of the pancreas ☐

329. On Figure B.26 arrow H is pointing to the:

> **a.** Gallbladder ☐
> **b.** Abdominal aorta ☐
> **c.** Right kidney ☐
> **d.** Left kidney ☐
> **e.** Adrenal gland ☐

330. On Figure B.26 arrow I is pointing to the:

> **a.** Gallbladder ☐
> **b.** Abdominal aorta ☐
> **c.** Right kidney ☐
> **d.** Left kidney ☐
> **e.** Adrenal gland ☐

331. On Figure B.26 arrow J is pointing to the:

> **a.** Gallbladder ☐
> **b.** Abdominal aorta ☐
> **c.** Right kidney ☐
> **d.** Left kidney ☐
> **e.** Adrenal gland ☐

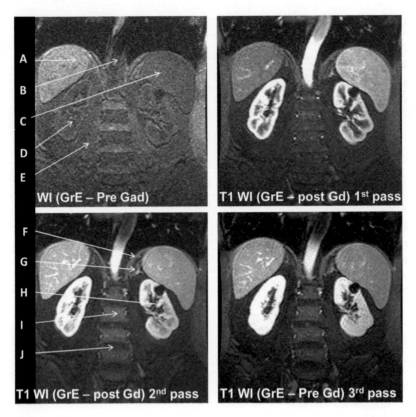

Figure B.27

332. On Figure B.27 arrow A is pointing to the:

   a. Liver ☐
   b. Abdominal aorta ☐
   c. Spleen ☐
   d. Gallbladder ☐
   e. Right kidney ☐

333. On Figure B.27 arrow B is pointing to the:

   a. Liver ☐
   b. Abdominal aorta ☐
   c. Spleen ☐
   d. Gallbladder ☐
   e. Right kidney ☐

334. On Figure B.27 arrow C is pointing to the:

> **a.** Liver ☐
> **b.** Abdominal aorta ☐
> **c.** Spleen ☐
> **d.** Gallbladder ☐
> **e.** Right kidney ☐

335. On Figure B.27 arrow D is pointing to the:

> **a.** Liver ☐
> **b.** Spleen ☐
> **c.** Gallbladder ☐
> **d.** Right kidney ☐
> **e.** Left kidney ☐

336. On Figure B.27 arrow E is pointing to the:

> **a.** Rectus abdominus muscles ☐
> **b.** Oblique muscles ☐
> **c.** Psoas muscle ☐
> **d.** Gluteal muscles ☐

337. On Figure B.27 arrow F is pointing to the:

> **a.** Cruz of the diaphragm ☐
> **b.** Adrenal gland ☐
> **c.** Right kidney ☐
> **d.** Left kidney ☐
> **e.** Pancreas ☐

338. On Figure B.27 arrow G is pointing to the:

> **a.** Cruz of the diaphragm ☐
> **b.** Adrenal gland ☐
> **c.** Right kidney ☐
> **d.** Left kidney ☐
> **e.** Pancreas ☐

339. On Figure B.27 arrow H is pointing to the:

    a. Cruz of the diaphragm ☐
    b. Adrenal gland ☐
    c. Right kidney ☐
    d. Left kidney ☐
    e. Pancreas ☐

340. On Figure B.27 arrow I is pointing to the:

    a. Rectus abdominus muscles ☐
    b. Oblique muscles ☐
    c. Psoas muscle ☐
    d. Lumbar vertebral body ☐
    e. Intervertebral disk ☐

341. On Figure B.27 arrow J is pointing to the:

    a. Rectus abdominus muscles ☐
    b. Oblique muscles ☐
    c. Psoas muscle ☐
    d. Lumbar vertebral body ☐
    e. Intervertebral disk ☐

Dynamic Enhanced Liver

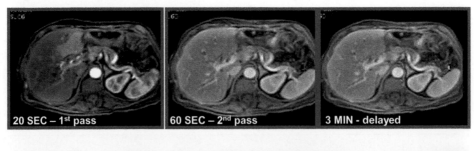

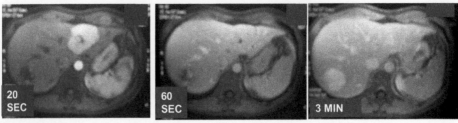

Figure B.28

342. On Figure B.28 shows images during various phases of contrast enhancement, including early (arterial – first pass), intermediate (cortico-venous phase – second pass), and delayed phases (third pass). Arterial phase imaging demonstrates all of the following characteristics EXCEPT:

a. Spleen is hyperintense to (brighter than) liver ☐
b. Spleen is "mottled" or "marbled" enhancement ☐
c. Only the cortex of the kidneys is enhanced ☐
d. The spleen and liver have the same signal intensity (isointense) ☐

343. Figure B.28 shows images during various phases of contrast enhancement. Most liver cancers are "arterially fed" and therefore are visualized on:

a. First-pass images ☐
b. Second-pass images ☐
c. Delayed images ☐
d. All phases ☐

344. Figure B.28 shows images during various phases of contrast enhancement. Hemangiomas are "benign" lesions (typically watch and wait lesions) that are venous fed, and therefore are visualized on:

a. First-pass images ☐
b. Second-pass images ☐
c. Delayed images ☐
d. All phases ☐

345. Patient positioning for abdominal MR images includes all of the following positions EXCEPT:

a. Supine, head first within the head coil ☐
b. Supine, head first within the torso array coil ☐
c. Supine, feet first within the torso array coil ☐
d. Prone, feet first within the torso array coil ☐

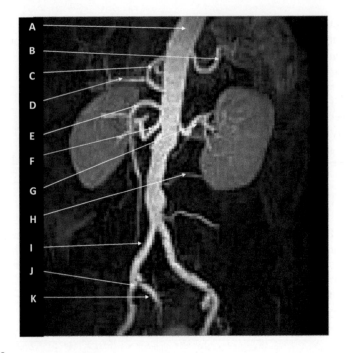

Figure B.29

346. On Figure B.29 arrow A is pointing to the:

    a. Abdominal aorta ☐
    b. Celiac artery ☐
    c. Splenic artery ☐
    d. Hepatic artery ☐
    e. Inferior vena cava (IVC) ☐

347. On Figure B.29 arrow B is pointing to the:

    a. Celiac artery ☐
    b. Splenic artery ☐
    c. Hepatic artery ☐
    d. Superior mesenteric artery ☐
    e. Spinal artery ☐

348. On Figure B.29 arrow C is pointing to the:

a. Celiac artery ☐
b. Splenic artery ☐
c. Hepatic artery ☐
d. Superior mesenteric artery ☐
e. Spinal artery ☐

349. On Figure B.29 arrow D is pointing to the:

a. Abdominal aorta ☐
b. Celiac artery ☐
c. Splenic artery ☐
d. Hepatic artery ☐
e. Superior mesenteric artery ☐

350. On Figure B.29 arrow E is pointing to the:

a. Celiac artery ☐
b. Splenic artery ☐
c. Hepatic artery ☐
d. Superior mesenteric artery ☐
e. Internal iliac artery ☐

351. On Figure B.29 arrow F is pointing to the:

a. Superior mesenteric artery ☐
b. Right renal artery ☐
c. Left renal artery ☐
d. Spinal artery ☐
e. Femoral artery ☐

352. On Figure B.29 arrow G is pointing to the:

a. Hepatic artery ☐
b. Superior mesenteric artery ☐
c. Right renal artery ☐
d. Left renal artery ☐

353. On Figure B.29 arrow H is pointing to the:

    a. Splenic artery ☐

    b. Right renal artery ☐

    c. Left renal artery ☐

    d. Spinal artery ☐

    e. Common iliac artery ☐

354. On Figure B.29 arrow I is pointing to the:

    a. Abdominal aorta ☐

    b. Celiac artery ☐

    c. Common iliac artery ☐

    d. Internal iliac artery ☐

    e. External iliac artery ☐

355. On Figure B.29 arrow J is pointing to the:

    a. Common iliac artery ☐

    b. Internal iliac artery ☐

    c. External iliac artery ☐

    d. Femoral artery ☐

356. On Figure B.29 arrow K is pointing to the:

    a. Spinal artery ☐

    b. Common iliac artery ☐

    c. Internal iliac artery ☐

    d. External iliac artery ☐

    e. Femoral artery ☐

357. Vascular imaging of the (arterial) abdominal vasculature (Figure B.29) is typically acquired with:

    a. 2D TOF MRA ☐

    b. 3D TOF MRA ☐

    c. 2D OC MRA ☐

    d. 3D PC MRA ☐

    e. Contrast-enhanced (CE) MRA ☐

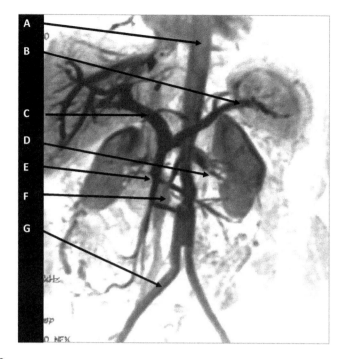

Figure B.30

358. On Figure B.30 arrow A is pointing to the:

    a. Abdominal aorta ☐
    b. Inferior vena cava ☐
    c. Femoral vein ☐
    d. Portal vein ☐
    e. Iliac artery ☐

359. On Figure B.30 arrow B is pointing to the:

    a. Femoral vein ☐
    b. Portal vein ☐
    c. Splenic vein ☐
    d. Renal vein ☐
    e. Superior mesenteric vein ☐

360. On Figure B.30 arrow C is pointing to the:

    a. Femoral vein ☐
    b. Portal vein ☐
    c. Splenic vein ☐
    d. Renal vein ☐
    e. Superior mesenteric vein ☐

361. On Figure B.30 arrow D is pointing to the:

    a. Portal vein ☐
    b. Splenic vein ☐
    c. Renal vein ☐
    d. Superior mesenteric vein ☐

362. On Figure B.30 arrow E is pointing to the:

    a. Portal vein ☐
    b. Splenic vein ☐
    c. Renal vein ☐
    d. Superior mesenteric vein ☐
    e. Iliac artery ☐

363. On Figure B.30 arrow F is pointing to the:

    a. Abdominal aorta ☐
    b. Inferior vena cava ☐
    c. Femoral vein ☐
    d. Portal vein ☐
    e. Iliac artery ☐

364. On Figure B.30 arrow G is pointing to the:

    a. Abdominal aorta ☐
    b. Inferior vena cava ☐
    c. Femoral vein ☐
    d. Portal vein ☐
    e. Iliac artery ☐

365. Vascular imaging of the (venous) abdominal vasculature (Figure B.30) is typically acquired with:

a. 2D TOF MRA

b. 3D TOF MRA

c. 2D OC MRA

d. 3D PC MRA

e. Contrast-enhanced (CE) MRA – delayed

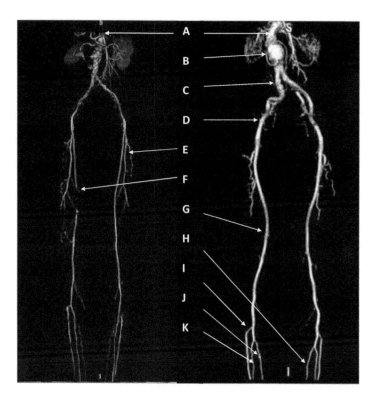

Figure B.31

366. Figure B.31 illustrates vascular imaging of the abdominal vasculature and runoff. This acquisition is acquired with dynamic contrast enhancement and:

a. Stationary table placement

b. Table stepping from the abdomen down to the legs

c. Table stepping from the legs up to the abdomen

d. With no specific table movement

367. On Figure B.31 arrow A is pointing to the:

> **a.** Abdominal aorta ☐
> **b.** Common iliac artery ☐
> **c.** Internal iliac artery ☐
> **d.** External iliac artery ☐

368. On Figure B.31 arrow B is pointing to the:

> **a.** Abdominal aorta ☐
> **b.** Abdominal aortic aneurysm ☐
> **c.** Common iliac artery ☐
> **d.** Internal iliac artery ☐

369. On Figure B.31 arrow C is pointing to the:

> **a.** Abdominal aorta ☐
> **b.** Common iliac artery ☐
> **c.** Internal iliac artery ☐
> **d.** External iliac artery ☐
> **e.** Femoral artery ☐

370. On Figure B.31 arrow D is pointing to the:

> **a.** Common iliac artery ☐
> **b.** Internal iliac artery ☐
> **c.** External iliac artery ☐
> **d.** Femoral artery ☐

371. On Figure B.31 arrow E is pointing to the:

> **a.** Common iliac artery ☐
> **b.** Internal iliac artery ☐
> **c.** External iliac artery ☐
> **d.** Common femoral artery ☐
> **e.** Superficial femoral artery ☐

372. On Figure B.31 arrow F is pointing to the:

> **a.** Common iliac artery ☐
> **b.** Vascular occlusion ☐
> **c.** Femoral artery ☐
> **d.** Popliteal artery ☐

373. On Figure B.31 arrow G is pointing to the:

- **a.** Popliteal artery ☐
- **b.** Anterior tibialis artery ☐
- **c.** Posterior tibialis artery ☐
- **d.** Peroneus brevus artery ☐

374. On Figure B.31 arrow H is pointing to the:

- **a.** Popliteal artery ☐
- **b.** Anterior tibialis artery ☐
- **c.** Posterior tibialis artery ☐
- **d.** Peroneus brevus artery ☐

375. On Figure B.31 arrow I is pointing to the:

- **a.** Popliteal artery ☐
- **b.** Anterior tibialis artery ☐
- **c.** Posterior tibialis artery ☐
- **d.** Peroneus brevus artery ☐

376. On Figure B.31 arrow J is pointing to the:

- **a.** Popliteal artery ☐
- **b.** Anterior tibialis artery ☐
- **c.** Posterior tibialis artery ☐
- **d.** Peroneus brevus artery ☐

377. On Figure B.31 arrow K is pointing to the:

- **a.** Popliteal artery ☐
- **b.** Anterior tibialis artery ☐
- **c.** Posterior tibialis artery ☐
- **d.** Peroneus brevus artery ☐

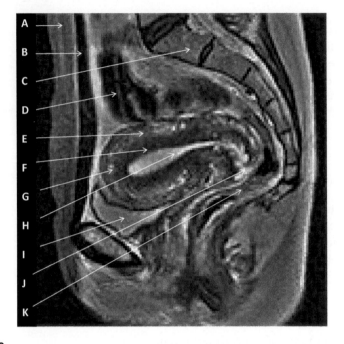

Figure B.32

378. On Figure B.32 arrow A is pointing to the:

- **a.** Subcutaneous fat ☐
- **b.** Rectus abdominus muscles ☐
- **c.** Oblique muscles ☐
- **d.** Lumbar spine ☐
- **e.** Sacrum ☐

379. On Figure B.32 arrow B is pointing to the:

- **a.** Subcutaneous fat ☐
- **b.** Rectus abdominus muscles ☐
- **c.** Oblique muscles ☐
- **d.** Lumbar spine ☐

380. On Figure B.32 arrow C is pointing to the:

- **a.** Rectus abdominus muscles ☐
- **b.** Oblique muscles ☐
- **c.** Lumbar spine ☐
- **d.** Sacrum ☐

381. On Figure B.32 arrow D is pointing to the:

- **a.** Subcutaneous fat ☐
- **b.** Rectus abdominus muscles ☐
- **c.** Oblique muscles ☐
- **d.** Lumbar spine ☐
- **e.** Bowel ☐

382. On Figure B.32 arrow E is pointing to the:

- **a.** Fundus ☐
- **b.** Myometrium ☐
- **c.** Junctional zone ☐
- **d.** Endometrium ☐
- **e.** Cervix ☐

383. On Figure B.32 arrow F is pointing to the:

- **a.** Fundus ☐
- **b.** Myometrium ☐
- **c.** Junctional zone ☐
- **d.** Endometrium ☐
- **e.** Cervix ☐

384. On Figure B.32 arrow G is pointing to the:

- **a.** Fundus ☐
- **b.** Myometrium ☐
- **c.** Junctional zone ☐
- **d.** Endometrium ☐
- **e.** Cervix ☐

385. On Figure B.32 arrow H is pointing to the:

- **a.** Fundus ☐
- **b.** Myometrium ☐
- **c.** Junctional zone ☐
- **d.** Endometrium ☐
- **e.** Cervix ☐

386. On Figure B.32 arrow I is pointing to the:

    a. Fundus ☐

    b. Endometrium ☐

    c. Cervix ☐

    d. Bladder ☐

    e. Rectum ☐

387. On Figure B.32 arrow J is pointing to the:

    a. Uterus ☐

    b. Junctional zone ☐

    c. Endometrium ☐

    d. Cervix ☐

    e. Bladder ☐

388. On Figure B.32 arrow K is pointing to the:

    a. Uterus ☐

    b. Fundus ☐

    c. Cervix ☐

    d. Bladder ☐

    e. Rectum ☐

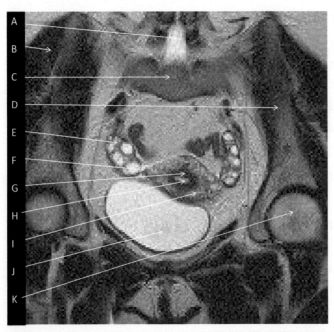

Figure B.33

389. On Figure B.33 arrow A is pointing to the:

- **a.** Spinal canal ☐
- **b.** Subcutaneous fat ☐
- **c.** Rectus abdominus muscles ☐
- **d.** Lumbar spine ☐
- **e.** Sacrum ☐

390. On Figure B.33 arrow B is pointing to the:

- **a.** Rectus abdominus muscles ☐
- **b.** Oblique muscles ☐
- **c.** Gluteal muscles ☐
- **d.** Fallopian tubes ☐
- **e.** Ovaries ☐

391. On Figure B.33 arrow C is pointing to the:

- **a.** Spinal canal ☐
- **b.** Subcutaneous fat ☐
- **c.** Lumbar spine ☐
- **d.** Sacrum ☐
- **e.** Bowel ☐

392. On Figure B.33 arrow D is pointing to the:

- **a.** Lumbar spine ☐
- **b.** Sacrum ☐
- **c.** Bowel ☐
- **d.** Ilium ☐
- **e.** Gluteal muscles ☐

393. On Figure B.33 arrow E is pointing to the:

- **a.** Uterus ☐
- **b.** Fundus ☐
- **c.** Cervix ☐
- **d.** Fallopian tubes ☐
- **e.** Ovaries ☐

394. On Figure B.33 arrow F is pointing to the:

> **a.** Uterus ☐
> **b.** Fundus ☐
> **c.** Cervix ☐
> **d.** Fallopian tubes ☐
> **e.** Ovaries ☐

395. On Figure B.33 arrow G is pointing to the:

> **a.** Fundus ☐
> **b.** Myometrium ☐
> **c.** Junctional zone ☐
> **d.** Endometrium ☐
> **e.** Cervix ☐

396. On Figure B.33 arrow H is pointing to the:

> **a.** Fundus ☐
> **b.** Myometrium ☐
> **c.** Junctional zone ☐
> **d.** Endometrium ☐
> **e.** Cervix ☐

397. On Figure B.33 arrow I is pointing to the:

> **a.** Fundus ☐
> **b.** Myometrium ☐
> **c.** Junctional zone ☐
> **d.** Endometrium ☐
> **e.** Cervix ☐

398. On Figure B.33 arrow J is pointing to the:

> **a.** Bowel ☐
> **b.** Uterus ☐
> **c.** Bladder ☐
> **d.** Rectum ☐

399. On Figure B.33 arrow K is pointing to the:

   a. Rectus abdominus muscles ☐
   b. Lumbar spine ☐
   c. Sacrum ☐
   d. Femoral head ☐

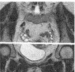

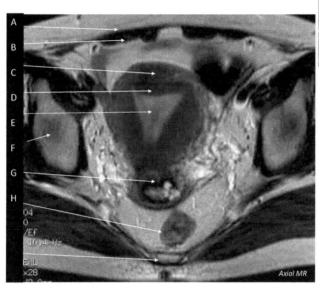

Figure B.34

400. On Figure B.34 arrow A is pointing to the:

   a. Subcutaneous fat ☐
   b. Rectus abdominus muscles ☐
   c. Oblique muscles ☐
   d. Lumbar spine ☐

401. On Figure B.34 arrow B is pointing to the:

   a. Subcutaneous fat ☐
   b. Rectus abdominus muscles ☐
   c. Oblique muscles ☐
   d. Lumbar spine ☐
   e. Sacrum ☐

402. On Figure B.34 arrow C is pointing to the:

   a. Uterus ☐
   b. Fundus ☐
   c. Myometrium ☐
   d. Junctional zone ☐
   e. Endometrium ☐

403. On Figure B.34 arrow D is pointing to the:

   a. Uterus ☐
   b. Fundus ☐
   c. Myometrium ☐
   d. Junctional zone ☐
   e. Endometrium ☐

404. On Figure B.34 arrow E is pointing to the:

   a. Fundus ☐
   b. Myometrium ☐
   c. Junctional zone ☐
   d. Endometrium ☐
   e. Cervix ☐

405. On Figure B.34 arrow F is pointing to the:

   a. Subcutaneous fat ☐
   b. Rectus abdominus muscles ☐
   c. Oblique muscles ☐
   d. Roof of the acetabulum ☐

406. On Figure B.34 arrow G is pointing to the:

   a. Fundus ☐
   b. Myometrium ☐
   c. Junctional zone ☐
   d. Endometrium ☐
   e. Cervix ☐

407. On Figure B.34 arrow H is pointing to the:

a. Rectus abdominus muscles ☐
b. Uterus ☐
c. Bladder ☐
d. Rectum ☐
e. Femoral head ☐

408. For female pelvic imaging, the best view for the evaluation of the uterus is the:

a. Sagittal ☐
b. Axial ☐
c. Coronal ☐
d. Oblique ☐

409. For female pelvic imaging, the best view for the evaluation of the ovaries is the:

a. Sagittal ☐
b. Axial ☐
c. Coronal ☐
d. Oblique ☐

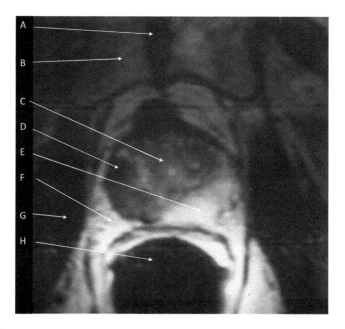

Figure B.35

410. On Figure B.35 arrow A is pointing to the:

> **a.** Symphysis pubis ☐
> **b.** Pubic bone ☐
> **c.** Rectum ☐
> **d.** Bladder ☐

411. On Figure B.35 arrow B is pointing to the:

> **a.** Symphysis pubis ☐
> **b.** Pubic bone ☐
> **c.** Central gland of the prostate ☐
> **d.** Rectum ☐

412. On Figure B.35 arrow C is pointing to the:

> **a.** Central gland of the prostate ☐
> **b.** Peripheral zone of the prostate (with cancer) ☐
> **c.** Peripheral zone of the prostate (without cancer) ☐
> **d.** Neurovascular bundle ☐
> **e.** Rectum ☐

413. On Figure B.35 arrow D is pointing to the:

> **a.** Central gland of the prostate ☐
> **b.** Peripheral zone of the prostate (with cancer) ☐
> **c.** Peripheral zone of the prostate (without cancer) ☐
> **d.** Neurovascular bundle ☐
> **e.** Rectum ☐

414. On Figure B.35 arrow E is pointing to the:

> **a.** Central gland of the prostate ☐
> **b.** Peripheral zone of the prostate (with cancer) ☐
> **c.** Peripheral zone of the prostate (without cancer) ☐
> **d.** Neurovascular bundle ☐
> **e.** Rectum ☐

415. On Figure B.35 arrow F is pointing to the:

a. Symphysis pubis ☐
b. Pubic bone ☐
c. Neurovascular bundle ☐
d. Obturator internus muscle ☐
e. Rectum ☐

416. On Figure B.35 arrow G is pointing to the:

a. Symphysis pubis ☐
b. Pubic bone ☐
c. Neurovascular bundle ☐
d. Obturator internus muscle ☐
e. Rectum ☐

417. On Figure B.35 arrow H is pointing to the:

a. Pubic bone ☐
b. Central gland of the prostate ☐
c. Rectum ☐
d. Bladder ☐
e. Prostatic urethra ☐

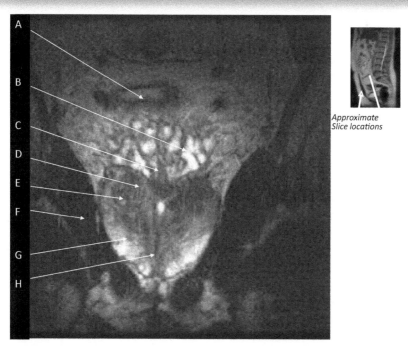

Approximate Slice locations

Figure B.36

418. On Figure B.36 arrow A is pointing to the:

a. Neurovascular bundle ☐
b. Rectum ☐
c. Bladder ☐
d. Seminal vesicles ☐

419. On Figure B.36 arrow B is pointing to the:

a. Seminal vesicles ☐
b. Vas deferens ☐
c. Prostatic urethra ☐
d. Base of the prostate ☐
e. Apex of the prostate ☐

420. On Figure B.36 arrow C is pointing to the:

a. Seminal vesicles ☐
b. Vas deferens ☐
c. Prostatic urethra ☐
d. Base of the prostate ☐
e. Apex of the prostate ☐

421. On Figure B.36 arrow D is pointing to the:

a. Central gland of the prostate ☐
b. Peripheral zone of the prostate (with cancer) ☐
c. Peripheral zone of the prostate (without cancer) ☐
d. Neurovascular bundle ☐

422. On Figure B.36 arrow E is pointing to the:

a. Neurovascular bundle ☐
b. Vas deferens ☐
c. Prostatic urethra ☐
d. Base of the prostate ☐
e. Apex of the prostate ☐

423. On Figure B.36 arrow F is pointing to the:

a. Symphysis pubis ☐
b. Pubic bone ☐
c. Obturator internus muscle ☐
d. Gluteal muscles ☐

424. On Figure B.36 arrow G is pointing to the:

a. Neurovascular bundle ☐
b. Vas deferens ☐
c. Prostatic urethra ☐
d. Base of the prostate ☐
e. Apex of the prostate ☐

425. On Figure B.36 arrow H is pointing to the:

a. Symphysis pubis ☐
b. Seminal vesicles ☐
c. Vas deferens ☐
d. Prostatic urethra ☐

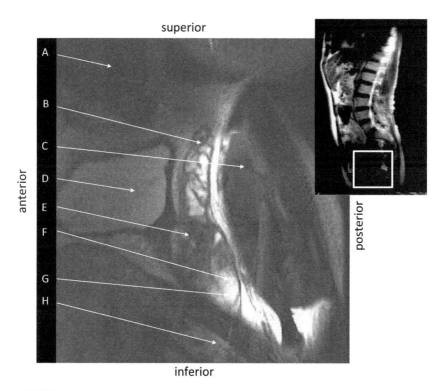

Figure B.37

426. On Figure B.37 arrow A is pointing to the:

> **a.** Bowel gas ☐
> **b.** Symphysis pubis ☐
> **c.** Pubic bone ☐
> **d.** Rectum ☐
> **e.** Bladder ☐

427. On Figure B.37 arrow B is pointing to the:

> **a.** Central gland of the prostate ☐
> **b.** Peripheral zone of the prostate ☐
> **c.** Neurovascular bundle ☐
> **d.** Seminal vesicles ☐

428. On Figure B.37 arrow C is pointing to the:

> **a.** Symphysis pubis ☐
> **b.** Rectum ☐
> **c.** Pubic bone ☐
> **d.** Bladder ☐

429. On Figure B.37 arrow D is pointing to the:

> **a.** Bowel gas ☐
> **b.** Bladder ☐
> **c.** Symphysis pubis ☐
> **d.** Pubic bone ☐
> **e.** Central gland of the prostate ☐
> **f.** Rectum ☐

430. On Figure B.37 arrow E is pointing to the:

> **a.** Vas deferens ☐
> **b.** Prostatic urethra ☐
> **c.** Base of the prostate ☐
> **d.** Apex of the prostate ☐

431. On Figure B.37 arrow F is pointing to the:

a. Central gland of the prostate ☐
b. Peripheral zone of the prostate ☐
c. Seminal vesicles ☐
d. Base of the prostate ☐
e. Apex of the prostate ☐

432. On Figure B.37 arrow G is pointing to the:

a. Symphysis pubis ☐
b. Central gland of the prostate ☐
c. Peripheral zone of the prostate ☐
d. Obturator internus muscle ☐
e. Apex of the prostate ☐

433. On Figure B.37 arrow H is pointing to the:

a. Symphysis pubis ☐
b. Central gland of the prostate ☐
c. Obturator internus muscle ☐
d. Gluteal muscles ☐

MRI of the musculoskeletal system

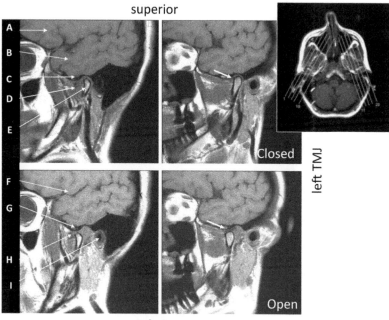

superior

inferior

Figure B.38

434. Since joints are situated "obliquely" within the body, MR imaging is acquired in the:

- **a.** Sagittal plane ☐
- **b.** Axial plane ☐
- **c.** Coronal plane ☐
- **d.** Oblique plane ☐

435. On Figure B.38 arrow A is pointing to the:

- **a.** Frontal lobe ☐
- **b.** Parietal lobe ☐
- **c.** Temporal lobe ☐
- **d.** Sylvian fissure ☐

436. On Figure B.38 arrow B is pointing to the:

- **a.** Frontal lobe ☐
- **b.** Parietal lobe ☐
- **c.** Temporal lobe ☐
- **d.** Sylvian fissure ☐

437. On Figure B.38 arrow C is pointing to the:

- **a.** Frontal bone ☐
- **b.** Parietal bone ☐
- **c.** Temporal bone ☐
- **d.** Condyle of the mandible ☐
- **e.** Mandible ☐

438. On Figure B.38 arrow D is pointing to the:

- **a.** Frontal bone ☐
- **b.** Parietal bone ☐
- **c.** Temporal bone ☐
- **d.** Meniscus ☐

439. On Figure B.38 arrow E is pointing to the:

- **a.** Sylvian fissure ☐
- **b.** Parietal bone ☐
- **c.** Temporal bone ☐
- **d.** Condyle of the mandible ☐
- **e.** Meniscus ☐

440. On Figure B.38 arrow F is pointing to the:

- **a.** Frontal lobe ☐
- **b.** Sylvian fissure ☐
- **c.** Parietal lobe ☐
- **d.** Temporal lobe ☐

441. On Figure B.38 arrow G is pointing to the:

- **a.** Eminence ☐
- **b.** Condyle of the mandible ☐
- **c.** Meniscus ☐
- **d.** Mandibular fossa ☐

442. On Figure B.38 arrow H is pointing to the:

- **a.** Meniscus ☐
- **b.** Eminence ☐
- **c.** Mandibular fossa ☐
- **d.** External auditory meatus (EAM) ☐

443. On Figure B.38 arrow I is pointing to the:

- **a.** Condyle of the mandible ☐
- **b.** Mandibular fossa ☐
- **c.** External auditory meatus (EAM) ☐
- **d.** Temporal bone (fossa) ☐
- **e.** Mandible ☐

444. Figure B.38 shows images of the TMJ for the evaluation of range of motion, whereby images are acquired:

- **a.** Open mouth only ☐
- **b.** Closed mouth only ☐
- **c.** Closed mouth and open mouth ☐
- **d.** With the mouth in the neutral position ☐

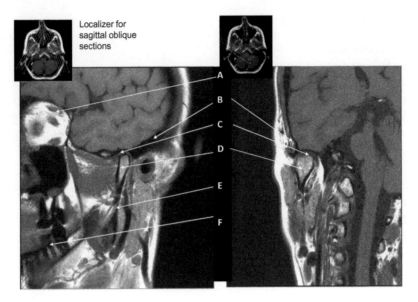

Figure B.39

445. TMJ imaging is acquired with oblique acquisition. The sagittal oblique images (Figure B.39, lower left) are acquired with slices:

    a. Perpendicular to the mandibular condyle ☐
    b. Parallel to the mandibular condyle ☐
    c. Along the parietal lobe ☐
    d. Perpendicular to the cervical spine ☐

446. TMJ imaging is acquired with oblique acquisition. The coronal oblique images (Figure B.39, lower right) are acquired with slices:

    a. Perpendicular to the mandibular condyle ☐
    b. Parallel to the mandibular condyle ☐
    c. Along the parietal lobe ☐
    d. Perpendicular to the cervical spine ☐

447. On Figure B.39 arrow A is pointing to the:

    a. Rectus muscles ☐
    b. Temporal lobe ☐
    c. Sylvian fissure ☐
    d. Condyle of the mandible ☐
    e. Meniscus ☐

448. On Figure B.39 arrow B is pointing to the:

a. Rectus muscles	☐
b. Parietal bone	☐
c. Temporal bone	☐
d. Condyle of the mandible	☐

449. On Figure B.39 arrow C is pointing to the:

a. Rectus muscles	☐
b. Temporal lobe	☐
c. Condyle of the mandible	☐
d. Meniscus	☐

450. On Figure B.39 arrow D is pointing to the:

a. Parietal bone	☐
b. Temporal bone	☐
c. Condyle of the mandible	☐
d. Mandibular fossa	☐

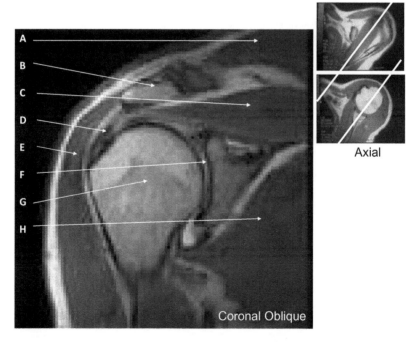

Axial

Coronal Oblique

Figure B.40

451. Shoulder imaging is acquired with oblique acquisition. The coronal oblique images (Figure B.40) with slices:

> **a.** Along the supraspinatus muscle (upper right – top) ☐
> **b.** Perpendicular to the glenoid fossa (upper right – bottom) ☐
> **c.** Straight coronal ☐
> **d.** a or b ☐

452. On Figure B.40 arrow A is pointing to the:

> **a.** Trapezius muscle ☐
> **b.** Deltoid muscle ☐
> **c.** Scaphoid subscapularis muscle ☐
> **d.** Subscapularis muscle ☐
> **e.** Biceps muscle ☐

453. On Figure B.40 arrow B is pointing to the:

> **a.** Humeral head ☐
> **b.** Acromion ☐
> **c.** Clavicle ☐
> **d.** Acromio-clavicular (AC) joint ☐

454. On Figure B.40 arrow C is pointing to the:

> **a.** Trapezius muscle ☐
> **b.** Deltoid muscle ☐
> **c.** Supraspinatus muscle ☐
> **d.** Infraspinatus muscle ☐
> **e.** Subscapularis muscle ☐

455. On Figure B.40 arrow D is pointing to the:

> **a.** Trapezius muscle ☐
> **b.** Deltoid muscle ☐
> **c.** Rotator cuff ☐
> **d.** Subscapularis muscle ☐

456. The structures that make up the rotator cuff include the:
   1. Trapezius muscle
   2. Supraspinatus muscle and tendon
   3. Infraspinatus muscle and tendon
   4. Teres minor muscle and tendon
   5. Subscapularis muscle and tendon
   6. Deltoid muscle

   a. 1 and 6   ☐
   b. 1, 2, 3, and 4   ☐
   c. 2, 3, 4, and 5   ☐
   d. 1, 2, 3, 4, 5, and 6   ☐

457. On Figure B.40 arrow E is pointing to the:

   a. Trapezius muscle   ☐
   b. Deltoid muscle   ☐
   c. Rotator cuff   ☐
   d. Biceps muscle   ☐

458. On Figure B.40 arrow F is pointing to the:

   a. Rotator cuff   ☐
   b. Glenoid fossa   ☐
   c. Acromio-clavicular (AC) joint   ☐
   d. Biceps muscle   ☐

459. On Figure B.40 arrow G is pointing to the:

   a. Rotator cuff   ☐
   b. Humeral head   ☐
   c. Acromion   ☐
   d. Clavicle   ☐
   e. Acromio-clavicular (AC) joint   ☐

460. On Figure B.40 arrow H is pointing to the:

   a. Trapezius muscle   ☐
   b. Supraspinatus muscle   ☐
   c. Infraspinatus muscle   ☐
   d. Teres minor muscle   ☐
   e. Subscapularis muscle   ☐

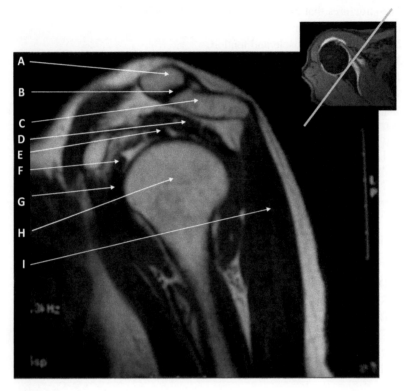

Figure B.41

461. On Figure B.41 arrow A is pointing to the:

    a. Acromion   ☐
    b. Clavicle   ☐
    c. Acromio-clavicular (AC) joint   ☐
    d. Humeral head   ☐

462. On Figure B.41 arrow B is pointing to the:

    a. Acromion   ☐
    b. Clavicle   ☐
    c. Acromio-clavicular (AC) joint   ☐
    d. Humeral head   ☐

463. On Figure B.41 arrow C is pointing to the:

a. Acromion ☐
b. Clavicle ☐
c. Acromio-clavicular (AC) joint ☐
d. Humeral head ☐

464. On Figure B.41 arrow D is pointing to the:

a. Supraspinatus tendon ☐
b. Infraspinatus tendon ☐
c. Teres minor tendon ☐
d. Subscapularis tendon ☐
e. Biceps muscle ☐

465. On Figure B.41 arrow E is pointing to the:

a. Supraspinatus tendon ☐
b. Infraspinatus tendon ☐
c. Teres minor tendon ☐
d. Subscapularis tendon ☐
e. Biceps muscle ☐

466. On Figure B.41 arrow F is pointing to the:

a. Supraspinatus tendon ☐
b. Infraspinatus tendon ☐
c. Teres minor tendon ☐
d. Subscapularis tendon ☐
e. Biceps muscle ☐

467. On Figure B.41 arrow G is pointing to the:

a. Supraspinatus tendon ☐
b. Infraspinatus tendon ☐
c. Teres minor tendon ☐
d. Subscapularis tendon ☐
e. Biceps muscle ☐

468. On Figure B.41 arrow H is pointing to the:

    a. Rotator cuff ☐
    b. Acromion ☐
    c. Clavicle ☐
    d. Humeral head ☐
    e. Biceps muscle ☐

469. On Figure B.41 arrow I is pointing to the:

    a. Trapezius muscle ☐
    b. Deltoid muscle ☐
    c. Subscapularis ☐
    d. Biceps muscle ☐

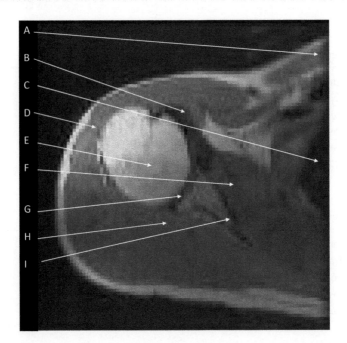

Figure B.42

470. On Figure B.42 arrow A is pointing to the:

    a. Pectoralis muscle ☐
    b. Subscapularis tendon ☐
    c. Lung ☐
    d. Deltoid muscle ☐

471. On Figure B.42 arrow B is pointing to the:

a. Pectoralis muscle ☐
b. Subscapularis tendon ☐
c. Lung ☐
d. Subscapularis muscle ☐
e. Glenoid fossa ☐

472. On Figure B.42 arrow C is pointing to the:

a. Pectoralis muscle ☐
b. Subscapularis tendon ☐
c. Lung ☐
d. Deltoid muscle ☐

473. On Figure B.42 arrow D is pointing to the:

a. Pectoralis muscle ☐
b. Subscapularis tendon ☐
c. Lung ☐
d. Deltoid muscle ☐
e. Subscapularis muscle ☐

474. On Figure B.42 arrow E is pointing to the:

a. Rotator cuff ☐
b. Humeral head ☐
c. Acromion ☐
d. Clavicle ☐
e. Scapula ☐

475. On Figure B.42 arrow F is pointing to the:

a. Trapezius muscle ☐
b. Subscapularis muscle ☐
c. Infraspinatus muscle ☐
d. Teres minor muscle ☐

476. On Figure B.42 arrow G is pointing to the:

a. Glenoid fossa ☐
b. Rotator cuff ☐
c. Acromio-clavicular (AC) joint ☐
d. Biceps muscle ☐

477. On Figure B.42 arrow H is pointing to the:

 a. Subscapularis muscle ☐
 b. Supraspinatus muscle ☐
 c. Infraspinatus muscle ☐
 d. Teres minor muscle ☐

478. On Figure B.42 arrow I is pointing to the:

 a. Scapula ☐
 b. Rotator cuff ☐
 c. Humeral head ☐
 d. Acromion ☐
 e. Clavicle ☐

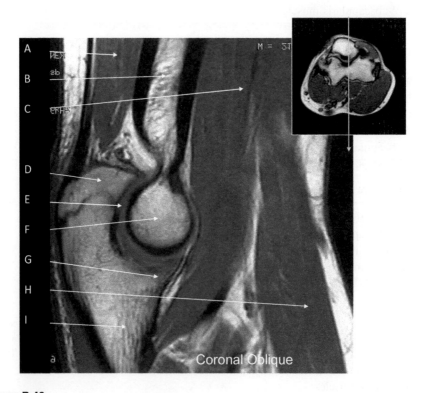

Figure B.43

479. On Figure B.43 arrow A is pointing to the:

> **a.** Biceps muscle ☐
> **b.** Triceps muscle ☐
> **c.** Brachioradialis muscles ☐
> **d.** Coronoid process ☐

480. On Figure B.43 arrow B is pointing to the:

> **a.** Humerus ☐
> **b.** Radius ☐
> **c.** Ulna ☐
> **d.** Capitellum ☐

481. On Figure B.43 arrow C is pointing to the:

> **a.** Biceps muscle ☐
> **b.** Triceps muscle ☐
> **c.** Brachioradialis muscles ☐
> **d.** Coronoid process ☐

482. On Figure B.43 arrow D is pointing to the:

> **a.** Olecranon process ☐
> **b.** Olecranon fossa ☐
> **c.** Humerus ☐
> **d.** Trochlea ☐
> **e.** Coronoid process ☐

483. On Figure B.43 arrow E is pointing to the:

> **a.** Olecranon process ☐
> **b.** Olecranon fossa ☐
> **c.** Humerus ☐
> **d.** Trochlea ☐
> **e.** Coronoid process ☐

484. On Figure B.43 arrow F is pointing to the:

> **a.** Olecranon process ☐
> **b.** Olecranon fossa ☐
> **c.** Humerus ☐
> **d.** Trochlea ☐
> **e.** Coronoid process ☐

485. On Figure B.43 arrow G is pointing to the:

a. Olecranon process ☐
b. Olecranon fossa ☐
c. Humerus ☐
d. Trochlea ☐
e. Coronoid process ☐

486. On Figure B.43 arrow H is pointing to the:

a. Biceps muscle ☐
b. Triceps muscle ☐
c. Brachioradialis muscles ☐
d. Coronoid process ☐

487. On Figure B.43 arrow I is pointing to the:

a. Olecranon process ☐
b. Olecranon fossa ☐
c. Humerus ☐
d. Ulna ☐
e. Radius ☐

488. Positioning for "optimal" elbow imaging can be "tricky" because of the elbow's location. For this reason positioning can be performed whereby the patient is:
1. Prone with the arm extended (over the head) within the extremity coil
2. Supine with the arm extended (over the head) within the extremity coil
3. Supine with the arm beside the patient (with a flex coil wrapped around the elbow)
4. Supine within the body coil

a. 1 only ☐
b. 1 and 2 only ☐
c. 2 and 3 only ☐
d. 1, 2, and 3 only ☐
e. 4 only ☐

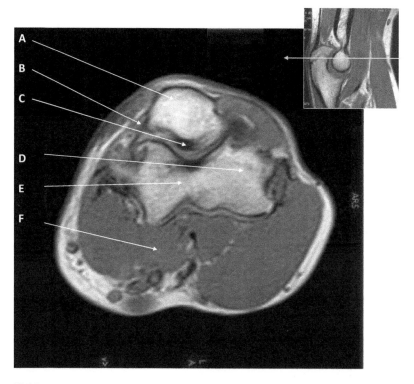

Figure B.44

489. On Figure B.44 arrow A is pointing to the:

    a. Olecranon process ☐
    b. Olecranon fossa ☐
    c. Flexor tendons ☐
    d. Extensor tendons ☐
    e. Brachioradialis muscles ☐

490. On Figure B.44 arrow B is pointing to the:

    a. Olecranon process ☐
    b. Olecranon fossa ☐
    c. Flexor tendons ☐
    d. Extensor tendons ☐
    e. Brachioradialis muscles ☐

491. Figure B.44 is displayed whereby the "top" of the image represents the _____ aspect of the elbow joint.

    a. Anterior ☐
    b. Posterior ☐
    c. Superior ☐
    d. Inferior ☐
    e. Right ☐

492. On Figure B.44 arrow C is pointing to the:

    a. Olecranon process ☐
    b. Olecranon fossa ☐
    c. Flexor tendons ☐
    d. Extensor tendons ☐
    e. Brachioradialis muscles ☐

493. On Figure B.44 arrow D is pointing to the:

    a. Olecranon process ☐
    b. Ulna ☐
    c. Brachioradialis muscles ☐
    d. Trochlea ☐
    e. Capitellum ☐

494. On Figure B.44 arrow E is pointing to the:

    a. Olecranon process ☐
    b. Ulna ☐
    c. Trochlea ☐
    d. Coronoid process ☐
    e. Capitellum ☐

495. On Figure B.44 arrow F is pointing to the:

    a. Flexor tendons ☐
    b. Extensor tendons ☐
    c. Brachioradialis muscles ☐
    d. Capitellum ☐

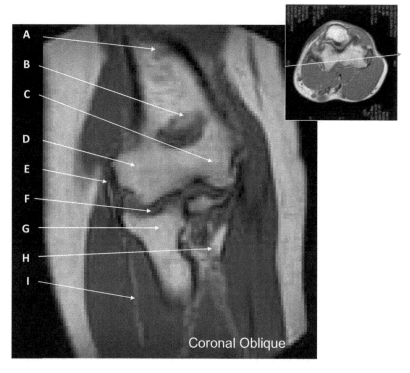

Figure B.45

496. On Figure B.45 arrow A is pointing to the:

a. Humerus	☐
b. Ulna	☐
c. Trochlea	☐
d. Radius	☐

497. On Figure B.45 arrow B is pointing to the:

a. Capitellum	☐
b. Trochlea	☐
c. Head of the radius	☐
d. Olecranon fossa	☐

498. On Figure B.45 arrow C is pointing to the:

a. Biceps muscle ☐
b. Humerus ☐
c. Ulna ☐
d. Trochlea ☐
e. Capitellum ☐

499. On Figure B.45 arrow D is pointing to the:

a. Capitellum ☐
b. Trochlea ☐
c. Head of the radius ☐
d. Ulna ☐

500. On Figure B.45 arrow E is pointing to the:

a. Biceps tendon ☐
b. Triceps tendon ☐
c. Lateral collateral ligament ☐
d. Head of the radius ☐
e. Capitellum ☐

501. On Figure B.45 arrow F is pointing to the:

a. Radio-ulnar joint ☐
b. Humero-radial joint ☐
c. Lateral collateral ligaments ☐
d. Head of the radius ☐
e. Capitellum ☐

502. On Figure B.45 arrow G is pointing to the:

a. Humerus ☐
b. Ulna ☐
c. Trochlea ☐
d. Coronoid process ☐
e. Head of the radius ☐

503. On Figure B.45 arrow H is pointing to the:

a. Humerus ☐
b. Ulna ☐
c. Trochlea ☐
d. Head of the radius ☐
e. Capitellum ☐

504. On Figure B.45 arrow I is pointing to the:

a. Biceps muscle ☐
b. Triceps muscle ☐
c. Brachioradialis muscles ☐
d. Capitellum ☐

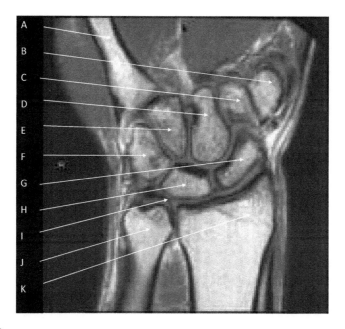

Figure B.46

505. On Figure B.46 arrow A is pointing to the:

a. Carpal tunnel ☐
b. Metacarpal ☐
c. Distal radius ☐
d. Distal ulna ☐

506. On Figure B.46 arrow B is pointing to the:

- **a.** Trapezium ☐
- **b.** Trapezoid ☐
- **c.** Capatate ☐
- **d.** Hammate ☐
- **e.** Triangular fibrocartilage complex (TFCC) ☐

507. On Figure B.46 arrow C is pointing to the:

- **a.** Trapezium ☐
- **b.** Trapezoid ☐
- **c.** Capatate ☐
- **d.** Hammate ☐
- **e.** Triangular fibrocartilage complex (TFCC) ☐

508. On Figure B.46 arrow D is pointing to the:

- **a.** Trapezium ☐
- **b.** Trapezoid ☐
- **c.** Capatate ☐
- **d.** Hammate ☐
- **e.** Triangular fibrocartilage complex (TFCC) ☐

509. On Figure B.46 arrow E is pointing to the:

- **a.** Trapezium ☐
- **b.** Trapezoid ☐
- **c.** Capatate ☐
- **d.** Hammate ☐
- **e.** TFCC ☐

510. On Figure B.46 arrow F is pointing to the:

- **a.** Scaphoid (navicular) ☐
- **b.** Lunate ☐
- **c.** Triquetrium ☐
- **d.** Pisiform ☐
- **e.** Trapezium ☐

511. On Figure B.46 arrow G is pointing to the:

    a. Scaphoid (navicular) ☐
    b. Lunate ☐
    c. Triquetrium ☐
    d. Pisiform ☐
    e. Trapezium ☐

512. On Figure B.46 arrow H is pointing to the:

    a. Scaphoid (navicular) ☐
    b. Lunate ☐
    c. Triquetrium ☐
    d. Pisiform ☐
    e. Trapezium ☐

513. On Figure B.46 arrow I is pointing to the:

    a. Scaphoid (navicular) ☐
    b. Hammate ☐
    c. Triangular fibrocartilage complex (TFCC) ☐
    d. Carpal tunnel ☐
    e. Distal radius ☐
    f. Distal ulna ☐

514. On Figure B.46 arrow J is pointing to the:

    a. Triangular fibrocartilage complex (TFCC) ☐
    b. Carpal tunnel ☐
    c. Distal radius ☐
    d. Distal ulna ☐

515. On Figure B.46 arrow K is pointing to the:

    a. Triangular fibrocartilage complex (TFCC) ☐
    b. Carpal tunnel ☐
    c. Distal radius ☐
    d. Distal ulna ☐

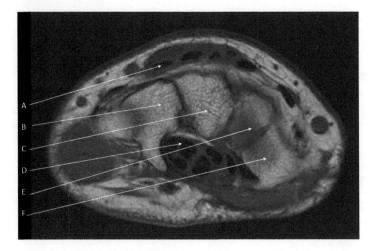

Figure B.47

516. On Figure B.47 arrow A is pointing to the:

> **a.** Flexor tendons ☐
> **b.** Extensor tendons ☐
> **c.** Carpal tunnel ☐
> **d.** Median nerve ☐

517. On Figure B.47 arrow is pointing to the:

> **a.** Trapezium ☐
> **b.** Trapezoid ☐
> **c.** Capatate ☐
> **d.** Hammate ☐

518. On Figure B.47 arrow C is pointing to the:

> **a.** Trapezium ☐
> **b.** Trapezoid ☐
> **c.** Capatate ☐
> **d.** Hammate ☐

519. On Figure B.47 arrow D is pointing to the:

> **a.** Flexor tendons ☐
> **b.** Extensor tendons ☐
> **c.** Carpal tunnel ☐
> **d.** Median nerve ☐

520. On Figure B.47 arrow E is pointing to the:

    a. Trapezium ☐
    b. Trapezoid ☐
    c. Capatate ☐
    d. Hammate ☐

521. On Figure B.47 arrow F is pointing to the:

    a. Trapezium ☐
    b. Trapezoid ☐
    c. Capatate ☐
    d. Hammate ☐

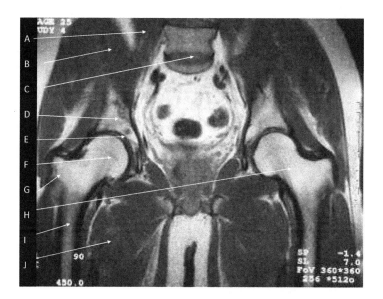

Figure B.48

522. To evaluate the hip joints, patient should be positioned whereby the:

    a. Feet are externally rotated ☐
    b. Feet are internally rotated ☐
    c. Feet are in the neutral position ☐
    d. Feet are turned toward the hip of interest ☐

523. On Figure B.48 arrow A is pointing to the:

> **a.** Psoas muscle ☐
> **b.** Iliacus muscle ☐
> **c.** Quadriceps muscle ☐
> **d.** Rectus abdominus muscles ☐
> **e.** Gluteal muscles ☐

524. On Figure B.48 arrow B is pointing to the:

> **a.** Psoas muscle ☐
> **b.** Iliacus muscle ☐
> **c.** Quadriceps muscle ☐
> **d.** Rectus abdominus muscles ☐
> **e.** Gluteal muscles ☐

525. On Figure B.48 arrow C is pointing to the:

> **a.** Lumbar vertebral body ☐
> **b.** Intervertebral disk ☐
> **c.** Sacrum ☐
> **d.** Rectus abdominus muscles ☐
> **e.** Gluteal muscles ☐

526. On Figure B.48 arrow D is pointing to the:

> **a.** Ilium ☐
> **b.** Acetabulum ☐
> **c.** Femoral head ☐
> **d.** Femoral neck ☐
> **e.** Greater trochantor ☐

527. On Figure B.48 arrow E is pointing to the:

> **a.** Ilium ☐
> **b.** Acetabulum ☐
> **c.** Femoral head ☐
> **d.** Femoral neck ☐
> **e.** Greater trochantor ☐

528. On Figure B.48 arrow F is pointing to the:

a. Ilium ☐
b. Acetabulum ☐
c. Femoral head ☐
d. Femoral neck ☐
e. Greater trochantor ☐

529. On Figure B.48 arrow G is pointing to the:

a. Ilium ☐
b. Acetabulum ☐
c. Femoral head ☐
d. Femoral neck ☐
e. Greater trochantor ☐

530. On Figure B.48 arrow H is pointing to the:

a. Ilium ☐
b. Acetabulum ☐
c. Femoral head ☐
d. Femoral neck ☐
e. Greater trochantor ☐

531. On Figure B.48 arrow I is pointing to the:

a. Femur ☐
b. Acetabulum ☐
c. Femoral head ☐
d. Femoral neck ☐
e. Greater trochantor ☐

532. On Figure B.48 arrow J is pointing to the:

a. Psoas muscle ☐
b. Iliacus muscle ☐
c. Quadriceps muscle ☐
d. Rectus abdominus muscles ☐
e. Gluteal muscles ☐

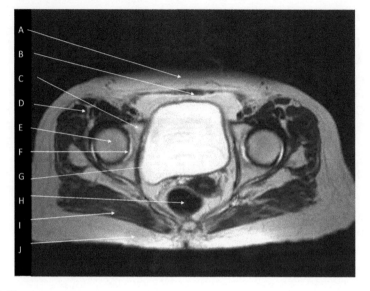

Figure B.49

533. On Figure B.49 arrow A is pointing to the:

    a. Psoas muscle ☐
    b. Subcutaneous fat ☐
    c. Rectus abdominus muscles ☐
    d. Gluteal muscles ☐

534. On Figure B.49 arrow B is pointing to the:

    a. Psoas muscle ☐
    b. Subcutaneous fat ☐
    c. Rectus abdominus muscles ☐
    d. Gluteal muscles ☐

535. On Figure B.49 arrow C is pointing to the:

    a. Ichium ☐
    b. Acetabulum ☐
    c. Iliac wing ☐
    d. Femoral head ☐
    e. Psoas muscle ☐

536. On Figure B.49 arrow D is pointing to the:

- **a.** Psoas muscle ☐
- **b.** Iliacus muscle ☐
- **c.** Quadriceps muscle ☐
- **d.** Rectus abdominus muscles ☐
- **e.** Gluteal muscles ☐

537. On Figure B.49 arrow E is pointing to the:

- **a.** Ichium ☐
- **b.** Acetabulum ☐
- **c.** Iliac wing ☐
- **d.** Femoral head ☐
- **e.** Psoas muscle ☐

538. On Figure B.49 arrow F is pointing to the:

- **a.** Ichium ☐
- **b.** Acetabulum ☐
- **c.** Iliac wing ☐
- **d.** Femoral head ☐

539. On Figure B.49 arrow G is pointing to the:

- **a.** Bladder ☐
- **b.** Rectum ☐
- **c.** Subcutaneous fat ☐
- **d.** Rectus abdominus muscles ☐
- **e.** Gluteal muscles ☐

540. On Figure B.49 arrow H is pointing to the:

- **a.** Bladder ☐
- **b.** Rectum ☐
- **c.** Subcutaneous fat ☐
- **d.** Rectus abdominus muscles ☐
- **e.** Gluteal muscles ☐

541. On Figure B.49 arrow I is pointing to the:

a. Psoas muscle ☐
b. Iliacus muscle ☐
c. Rectus abdominus muscles ☐
d. Gluteal muscles ☐

542. On Figure B.49 arrow J is pointing to the:

a. Rectum ☐
b. Subcutaneous fat ☐
c. Rectus abdominus muscles ☐
d. Gluteal muscles ☐

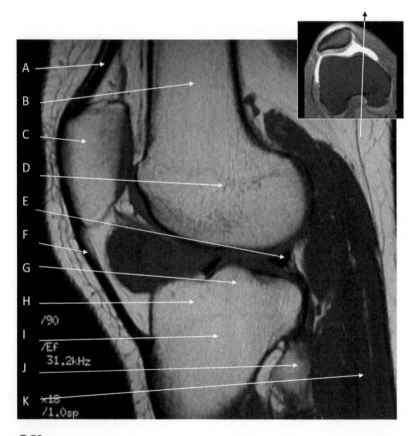

Figure B.50

543. On Figure B.50 arrow A is pointing to the:

> **a.** Quadriceps tendon ☐
> **b.** Patellar ligament ☐
> **c.** Medial collateral ligament ☐
> **d.** Lateral collateral ligament ☐
> **e.** Medial retinaculum ☐
> **f.** Lateral retinaculum ☐

544. On Figure B.50 arrow B is pointing to the:

> **a.** Femur ☐
> **b.** Patella ☐
> **c.** Femoral condyle ☐
> **d.** Tibial plateau ☐
> **e.** Tibial spine ☐

545. On Figure B.50 arrow C is pointing to the:

> **a.** Femur ☐
> **b.** Patella ☐
> **c.** Femoral condyle ☐
> **d.** Tibial plateau ☐
> **e.** Tibial spine ☐

546. On Figure B.50 arrow D is pointing to the:

> **a.** Femur ☐
> **b.** Patella ☐
> **c.** Femoral condyle ☐
> **d.** Tibial plateau ☐
> **e.** Tibial spine ☐

547. On Figure B.50 arrow E is pointing to the:

> **a.** Posterior horn of the lateral meniscus ☐
> **b.** Posterior horn of the medial meniscus ☐
> **c.** Anterior horn of the lateral meniscus ☐
> **d.** Anterior horn of the medial meniscus ☐

548. On Figure B.50 arrow F is pointing to the:

    a. Quadriceps tendon ☐
    b. Patellar ligament ☐
    c. Medial collateral ligament ☐
    d. Lateral collateral ligament ☐
    e. Medial retinaculum ☐
    f. Lateral retinaculum ☐

549. On Figure B.50 arrow G is pointing to the:

    a. Femur ☐
    b. Patella ☐
    c. Femoral condyle ☐
    d. Tibial plateau ☐
    e. Tibial spine (eminence) ☐

550. On Figure B.50 arrow H is pointing to the:

    a. Femur ☐
    b. Patella ☐
    c. Femoral condyle ☐
    d. Tibial plateau ☐
    e. Tibial spine ☐

551. On Figure B.50 arrow I is pointing to the:

    a. Femur ☐
    b. Patella ☐
    c. Tibia ☐
    d. Fibula ☐

552. On Figure B.50 arrow J is pointing to the:

    a. Femur ☐
    b. Patella ☐
    c. Tibia ☐
    d. Fibula ☐

553. On Figure B.50 arrow K is pointing to the:

   a. Quadriceps muscle ☐
   b. Triceps muscle ☐
   c. Gastrocnemius muscle ☐
   d. Medial collateral ligament ☐
   e. Lateral collateral ligament ☐
   f. Medial retinaculum ☐
   g. Lateral retinaculum ☐

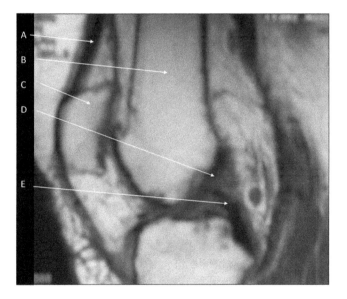

Figure B.51

554. To evaluate the anterior cruciate ligament (ACL) within the knee, the patient should be positioned whereby the:

   a. Feet are externally rotated ☐
   b. Feet are internally rotated ☐
   c. Feet are in the neutral position ☐
   d. Feet are turned toward the hip of interest ☐

555. The best view or views for the evaluation of the anterior cruciate ligament (ACL) include:
1. Sagittal
2. Axial
3. Coronal
4. Oblique

    a. 1 only
    b. 1 and 2 only
    c. 1 and 4 only
    d. 1, 2, and 3 only
    e. 4 only

556. On Figure B.51 arrow A is pointing to the:

    a. Quadriceps tendon
    b. Patellar ligament
    c. Medial collateral ligament
    d. Lateral collateral ligament
    e. Medial retinaculum
    f. Lateral retinaculum

557. On Figure B.51 arrow B is pointing to the:

    a. Femur
    b. Patella
    c. Femoral condyle
    d. Tibial plateau
    e. Tibial spine

558. On Figure B.51 arrow C is pointing to the:

    a. Femur
    b. Patella
    c. Femoral condyle
    d. Tibial plateau
    e. Tibial spine

559. On Figure B.51 arrow D is pointing to the:

    a. Anterior cruciate ligament (ACL)   □
    b. Posterior cruciate ligament (PCL)   □
    c. Quadriceps tendon   □
    d. Patellar ligament   □
    e. Lateral retinaculum   □

560. On Figure B.51 arrow E is pointing to the:

    a. Anterior cruciate ligament (ACL)   □
    b. Posterior cruciate ligament (PCL)   □
    c. Quadriceps tendon   □
    d. Patellar ligament   □
    e. Lateral retinaculum   □

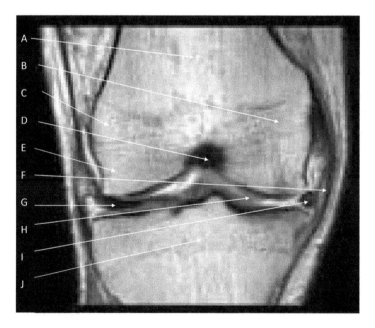

Figure B.52

561. On Figure B.52 arrow A is pointing to the:

a. Femur ☐
b. Patella ☐
c. Femoral condyle ☐
d. Medial epicondyle of the femur ☐
e. Lateral epicondyle of the femur ☐
f. Medial condyle of the femur ☐
g. Lateral condyle of the femur ☐

562. On Figure B.52 arrow B is pointing to the:

a. Patella ☐
b. Femoral condyle ☐
c. Medial epicondyle of the femur ☐
d. Lateral epicondyle of the femur ☐
e. Medial condyle of the femur ☐
f. Lateral condyle of the femur ☐

563. On Figure B.52 arrow C is pointing to the:

a. Patella ☐
b. Femoral condyle ☐
c. Medial epicondyle of the femur ☐
d. Lateral epicondyle of the femur ☐
e. Medial condyle of the femur ☐
f. Lateral condyle of the femur ☐

564. On Figure B.52 arrow D is pointing to the:

a. Intercondylar fossa ☐
b. Patella ☐
c. Femoral condyle ☐
d. Medial epicondyle of the femur ☐
e. Lateral epicondyle of the femur ☐
f. Medial condyle of the femur ☐
g. Lateral condyle of the femur ☐

565. On Figure B.52 arrow E is pointing to the:

  a. Patella □
  b. Femoral condyle □
  c. Medial epicondyle of the femur □
  d. Lateral epicondyle of the femur □
  e. Medial condyle of the femur □
  f. Lateral condyle of the femur □

566. On Figure B.52 arrow F is pointing to the:

  a. Medial collateral ligament □
  b. Lateral collateral ligament □
  c. Medial retinaculum □
  d. Lateral retinaculum □

567. On Figure B.52 arrow G is pointing to the:

  a. Anterior cruciate ligament (ACL) □
  b. Posterior cruciate ligament (PCL) □
  c. Lateral meniscus □
  d. Medial meniscus □

568. On Figure B.52 arrow H is pointing to the:

  a. Interarticular cartilage □
  b. Posterior horn of the lateral meniscus □
  c. Posterior horn of the medial meniscus □
  d. Anterior horn of the lateral meniscus □
  e. Anterior horn of the medial meniscus □

569. On Figure B.52 arrow I is pointing to the:

  a. Anterior cruciate ligament (ACL) □
  b. Posterior cruciate ligament (PCL) □
  c. Lateral meniscus □
  d. Medial meniscus □

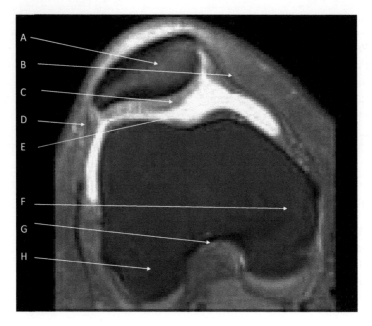

Figure B.53

570. On Figure B.53 arrow A is pointing to the:

> **a.** Patella ☐
> **b.** Femoral medial condyle ☐
> **c.** Femoral lateral condyle ☐
> **d.** Tibia ☐
> **e.** Fibula ☐

571. On Figure B.53 arrow B is pointing to the:

> **a.** Quadriceps tendon ☐
> **b.** Medial collateral ligament ☐
> **c.** Lateral collateral ligament ☐
> **d.** Medial retinaculum ☐
> **e.** Lateral retinaculum ☐

572. On Figure B.53 arrow C is pointing to the:

> **a.** Patello-femoral joint ☐
> **b.** Femoral medial condyle ☐
> **c.** Femoral lateral condyle ☐
> **d.** Tibia ☐
> **e.** Fibula ☐

573. On Figure B.53 arrow D is pointing to the:

    a. Quadriceps tendon ☐
    b. Medial collateral ligament ☐
    c. Lateral collateral ligament ☐
    d. Medial retinaculum ☐
    e. Lateral retinaculum ☐

574. On Figure B.53 arrow E is pointing to the:

    a. Meniscus ☐
    b. Fluid within the joint space ☐
    c. Patellar Ligament ☐
    d. Condyle ☐

575. On Figure B.53 arrow F is pointing to the:

    a. Intercondylar fossa ☐
    b. Femoral medial condyle ☐
    c. Femoral lateral condyle ☐
    d. Tibia ☐
    e. Fibula ☐

576. On Figure B.53 arrow G is pointing to the:

    a. Intercondylar fossa ☐
    b. Femoral medial condyle ☐
    c. Femoral lateral condyle ☐
    d. Tibia ☐
    e. Fibula ☐

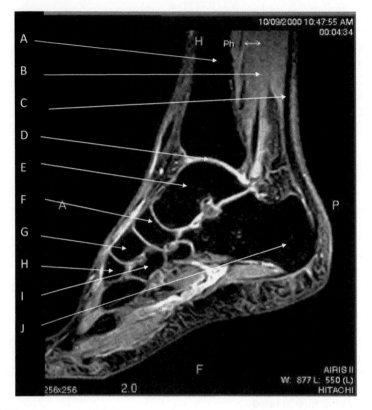

Figure B.54

577. On Figure B.54 arrow A is pointing to the:

   a. Tibia ☐
   b. Talus ☐
   c. Navicular ☐
   d. Calcaneus ☐
   e. Fibula ☐

578. On Figure B.54 arrow B is pointing to the:

   a. Gastrocnemius muscle ☐
   b. Achilles tendon ☐
   c. Tibio-talar joint ☐
   d. Talus ☐
   e. Navicular ☐

579. On Figure B.54 arrow C is pointing to the:

a. Gastrocnemius muscle ☐
b. Achilles tendon ☐
c. Tibio-talar joint ☐
d. Talus ☐
e. Navicular ☐

580. On Figure B.54 arrow D is pointing to the:

a. Gastrocnemius muscle ☐
b. Achilles tendon ☐
c. Tibio-talar joint ☐
d. Talus ☐
e. Navicular ☐

581. On Figure B.54 arrow E is pointing to the:

a. Gastrocnemius muscle ☐
b. Achilles tendon ☐
c. Tibio-talar joint ☐
d. Talus ☐
e. Navicular ☐

582. On Figure B.54 arrow F is pointing to the:

a. Talus ☐
b. Navicular ☐
c. Cuboid ☐
d. Calcaneus ☐
e. Plantar surface ☐

583. On Figure B.54 arrow G is pointing to the:

a. Talus ☐
b. Navicular ☐
c. Cuboid ☐
d. Calcaneus ☐
e. Plantar surface ☐

584. On Figure B.54 arrow H is pointing to the:

> **a.** Talus ☐
> **b.** Cuboid ☐
> **c.** Phalanx ☐
> **d.** Metatarsals ☐
> **e.** Tarsal tunnel ☐

585. On Figure B.54 arrow I is pointing to the:

> **a.** Navicular ☐
> **b.** Cuneiform ☐
> **c.** Cuboid ☐
> **d.** Calcaneus ☐
> **e.** Phalanx ☐

586. On Figure B.54 arrow J is pointing to the:

> **a.** Navicular ☐
> **b.** Cuboid ☐
> **c.** Calcaneus ☐
> **d.** Tarsal tunnel ☐
> **e.** Plantar surface ☐

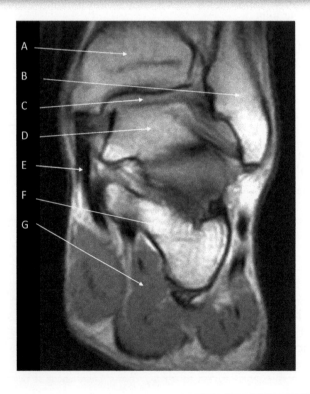

Figure B.55

587. On Figure B.55 arrow A is pointing to the:

a. Tibia ☐
b. Tibio-talar joint ☐
c. Talus ☐
d. Navicular ☐
e. Cuboid ☐

588. On Figure B.55 arrow B is pointing to the:

a. Tibia ☐
b. Fibula ☐
c. Talus ☐
d. Navicular ☐
e. Calcaneus ☐

589. On Figure B.55 arrow C is pointing to the:

a. Tibia ☐
b. Achilles tendon ☐
c. Tibio-talar joint ☐
d. Talus ☐

590. On Figure B.55 arrow D is pointing to the:

a. Tibia ☐
b. Talus ☐
c. Navicular ☐
d. Cuboid ☐
e. Calcaneus ☐

591. On Figure B.55 arrow E is pointing to the:

a. Medial collateral ligament ☐
b. Lateral collateral ligament ☐
c. Achilles tendon ☐
d. Tibio-talar joint ☐
e. Tarsal tunnel ☐
f. Plantar surface ☐

592. On Figure B.55 arrow F is pointing to the:

a. Tibia ☐
b. Navicular ☐
c. Cuboid ☐
d. Calcaneus ☐

593. On Figure B.55 arrow G is pointing to the:

    a. Tibio-talar joint   ☐
    b. Talus   ☐
    c. Metatarsals   ☐
    d. Tarsal tunnel   ☐
    e. Plantar surface   ☐

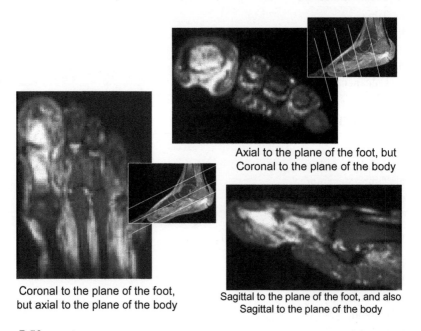

Axial to the plane of the foot, but
Coronal to the plane of the body

Coronal to the plane of the foot,
but axial to the plane of the body

Sagittal to the plane of the foot, and also
Sagittal to the plane of the body

Figure B.56

594. Figure B.56 shows examples of sagittal, axial, and coronal images of the foot. When the patient is positioned in the "anatomic man" position, whereby the patient is facing us, flat footed, the imaging planes vary whereby images acquired:

    a. Coronal to the plane of the body, create images axial to the plane of the foot   ☐
    b. Coronal to the plane of the body, create images coronal to the plane of the foot   ☐
    c. Axial to the plane of the body, create images axial to the plane of the foot   ☐
    d. Sagittal to the plane of the body, create images axial to the plane of the foot   ☐

Part B: Answers

1. **b**

2. **a**

   Contrast-enhanced MR images where fat is bright, water [or in this case cerebrospinal fluid (CSF)] appears dark, and gray matter is brighter than white matter are showing T1 characteristics. Such images are known as T1-weighted images whereby the image contrast is "heavily" in favor of T1 characteristics. For more questions on image contrast, refer to Part C.

3. **a**

   These images were acquired with a spin echo (SE) acquisition. T1WI (SE images) are acquired with a short TR (approximately 400–800 ms for brain imaging) and short TE (approximately 20 ms or below).

4. **c**

5. **d**

6. **b**

7. **b**

   Generally speaking, the brain is made up of gray and white matter, whereby the gray matter is located on the outer surface of the brain (known as the cortex) and the white matter is located within the brain. The hemispheres are also covered with gray matter. In this midline sagittal image of the brain, the parietal lobe is imaged in the mid-sagittal location, and therefore on the "midline, gray matter covering" of the brain tissue. Even though arrow B appears to point at an area where white matter would be, this is a mid-sagittal imaging section and the hemispheres are covered with gray matter.

8. **b**

9. **b**

10. **a**

    The corpus callosum is the only white matter structure to cross the midline. The anterior position is known as the genu and the posterior position is known as the splenium.

11. **a**

12. **c**

13. **a**

14. **b**

15. **c**

16. **b**

17. d

18. a

19. c

20. a

21. c

22. c

23. c

24. c

25. d

26. c

27. d

28. c

29. b

Generally speaking, the spinal cord is made up of gray and white matter, whereby the white matter fibers are located along the outer surface of the cord and the gray matter is within. The cord is essentially "inside-out" when compared to the brain. Since this is a midline section of the brain and spinal cord, the tissue defined by arrow O is within the cord, and therefore gray matter.

30. b

31. c

32. c

Metastatic disease tends to demonstrate delayed enhancement. For this reason, rapid imaging is not used when there is a suspicion of metastases. One contrast agent is approved for single dose followed by double dose, giving a total triple dose.

33. a

34. c

35. b

36. a

37. c

When imaging a patient with hemorrhagic lesions, the signal intensity of the lesion varies with the "relative age" of the bleed. If imaging is performed immediately after the hemorrhagic lesion has occurred (oxyhemoglobin), the blood is isointense with brain tissue. As time elapses, blood "breaks down" and oxyhemoglobin becomes deoxyhemoglobin. At this point, blood appears bright on T1WI and darker on T2WI. The next phase is the formation of methemoglobin. At this point blood appears bright on both T1WI and T2WI. Finally, hemaciderin (essentially iron) forms and this appears dark on T1WI and T2WI, as iron/metal would appear. For these reasons the radiologist can identify the relative age of the hemorrhagic lesion.

38. a

39. b

40. b

To evaluate structures within the body (particularly smaller structures within the head), the optimal imaging plane is the "view" that demonstrates the structure in "profile". The IACs are positioned bilaterally and run from the pons to the EAM (external auditory meatus). For this reason, the best views include the axial plane and the coronal plane. Bear in mind that imaging planes can vary with patient positioning. For example, if the patient is positioned obliquely and/or if the patient's head is hyper extended within the head coil, oblique images might be required to demonstrate the IAC's coronal or axial to the plane of the anatomy.

41. d

Inversion recovery imaging sequences rely on T1 relaxation. The TI (inversion time or time to inversion) allows time for T1 recovery to occur in the gray and white matter, while in the presence of the magnetic field. This phenomenon tends to enhance gray/white matter differences more than conventional spin echo T1-weighted images or spoiled gradient echoes. For this reason, IR sequences with TI times of approximaterly 600 ms (at 1.5 T) would be optimal for infant imaging (i.e. children under 1 year of age).

42. c

MR images can be acquired in sagittal, axial, coronal, or oblique imaging planes. Images can also be acquired with one of several image contrast characteristics, including T1WI [with and without contrast media (gadolinium)], T2WI (and T2* gradient echo acquisitions), PDWI, and FLAIR imaging. A typical brain protocol consists of a sagittal T1WI, axial T2WI, axial FLAIR or PDWI, and axial diffusion images.

Figure B.57 shows examples of sagittal T1WI, axial PDWI, axial FLAIR, and coronal T2WI images. The brain is made up primarily of gray matter and white matter. The gray matter "ribbons" (the brain's cortex) is typically located on the outer portion of the brain. White matter "fibers" are located on the inside of the brain. The exception is a group of structures known as the basal ganglia. These "islands" of gray matter are located within the brain. On T1WI, the fat is bright, water dark, and gray matter is brighter than white matter. On T2WI, the water is bright, fat darker, and white matter darker than gray matter. On PDWI, the fluid and fat are bright and the gray matter ribbons are brighter than white matter. On FLAIR images, the darkness of the brain structures is similar to that of PDWI (white matter darker than gray matter), fat is bright, and fluid is attenuated or suppressed. Compare the image contrast and imaging planes with those in Figures B.1–B.6.

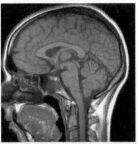

Midline Sagittal T1WI

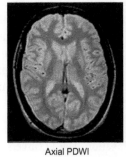

Axial PDWI

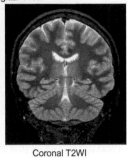

Axial FLAIR   Coronal T2WI

Figure B.57   Image contrast by MRI.

43. a

44. c

45. c

46. b

47. a

48. a

49. a

50. b

51. c

52. a

53. d

54. b

55. d

56. d

57. c

58. a

Depending upon the type of image acquired (T1WI, T2WI, PDWI, and/or FLAIR images), particular structures are brighter than (hyperintense) or darker than (hypointense) other structure on the image. For example, when T2WI are acquired, water is hyperintense to (brighter than) fat and brain tissue. On T1WI, water is hypointense to (darker than) fat and brain tissue. The white matter sheath consists of interwoven fat and protein; fat is brighter than gray matter on T1WI. Remember fat is bright on T1WI.

59. d

There are 12 cranial nerves that are visible on MR images. The seventh (acoustic or vestibulocochlear) and eighth (facial) cranial nerves run though the internal auditory canals and are often visible on high-resolution MR images. Regarding other cranial nerves commonly evaluated by MR imaging, the second cranial nerve is the optic nerve, the fifth is the trigeminal, and the 10th (vagus nerve) is the largest cranial nerve running from the brain to the diaphragm.

60. c

According to the ACR, typical brain protocols include sagittal T1WI, axial T2WI (FSE preferred if available; if not, SE), axial FLAIR (preferred if available) or PDWI, and diffusion imaging (preferred if available). Contrast-enhanced sequences are not always required, but can be added to the protocol for the evaluation of infection, infarction, inflammation, and/or neoplasm, in accordance with the institutional policy.

61. a

62. d

63. d

64. d

65. d

66. b

67. d

68. c

Diffusion imaging is performed with the use of echo planar imaging (T2* gradient echo acquisitions) and the application of "diffusion gradients". Diffusion gradients utilize the application of additional gradient pulses applied along the x, y, and z directions. The strength and duration of these diffusion gradient pulses is selected by a user-selectable parameter known as the "B" value. Tissues with "restricted" diffusion (like tissues in a new stroke or hyperacute infarct) appear bright on diffusion-weighted imaging. Even though there is intracellular and extracellular fluid associated with stroke, such lesions (new strokes) are not visualized on conventional FLAIR, PDWI, and/or T2WI.

69. b

70. d

The terms "landmark" and "centering" as used in MRI need to be differentiated. The term landmark is used when the patent is placed into the MR imager for their imaging procedure. For typical brain imaging, all patients are "landmarked" at the location of the nasion. This will "center" the head within isocenter of the imager for head imaging. When a particular pathologic condition or anatomic location is to be imaged, the slices are "centered" at the location of the pathology or anatomy of interest. In Figures B.2 and B.3, the concept of landmark was utilized for "general head imaging". The concept of "centering" was used for the evaluation of a patient with ""tinnitus" (ringing in the ears). For this reason, the slices should be "centered" to the external auditory meatus, the ears.

71. b

72. c

73. b

74. c

75. a

76. a

77. b

78. a

79. d

80. c

81. c

82. d

83. d

84. d

85. b

86. c

87. a

hyperintense = brighter than,
hypointense = darker than,
isointense = the same signal intensity as.

88. a

89. b

90. c

91. a

92. a

93. c

94. a

95. e

96. c

97. b

98. b

99. a

100. d

Tissues with short T1 relaxation times appear bright (hyperintense) on T1-weighted images. T1 relaxation is also known as T1 recovery, longitudinal recovery and/or spin lattice. Gadolinium is paramagnetic and therefore affects (shortens) the T1 relaxation times of tissues. For this reason, enhancing structures in the CNS (central nervous system / brain and spine), such as infection, infarction, inflammation, and/ or neoplasm (tumors), appear bright on T1WI.

Contrast media do not cross the "intact" blood–brain barrier (BBB) in MRI (or in CT). Gadolinium does, however, enhance normal anatomic structures that are located outside the BBB, these are said to be extra-axial. The normal structures that can demonstrate enhancement in MR images include: the pituitary gland (also known as the hypophysis), pituitary stalk (also known as the infundibulum), pineal gland, falx cerebri, slow flowing vessels [like the distal branches of arteries of the head and venous structures (known as dural sinuses)], choroid plexus (within the anterior and posterior horns of the lateral ventricles, and which produces CSF), sinus mucosa, and some facial muscles.

101. a

102. c

T1 and T2 relaxation times are inter-related whereby if the T1 time is affected (shortened) the T2 relaxation time is also affected (shortened). Tissues with short T2 relaxation times appear dark (hypointense) on T2-weighted images (particularly gradient echo T2* imaging). The MR images in Figure B.6 are displayed without and with contrast media. On T1WI, gadolinium shortens the T1 time (of the lesion), making the lesion appear bright on T1WI. On T2*WI, gadolinium shortens the T2* time, making the brain darker on T2*WI. Gadolinium is used for perfusion imaging of the brain. This technique is known as dynamic susceptibility-weighted imaging (DSWI). In this case, T2* echo planar imaging is performed rapidly, with multiple acquisitions acquired before, during, and after the administration of gadolinium. Regions of the brain that have normal blood supply will appear dark. Regions of the brain with limited blood supply (as the result of stroke) appear bright (as compared to the darkened regions of normal brain).

103. a

104. d

105. a

106. c

107. a

108. a

109. c

110. e

111. a

112. c

113. d

The vasculature within the brain is known as the "circle of Willis". On the axial view (Figure B.7) the image is displayed whereby the "top" of the image is the anterior (frontal lobe) of the brain, and the "bottom" is the posterior (occipital lobe). Remember, MR images (like radiographic images) are viewed whereby the right side of the image is the left of the patient (as if we are facing the patient on the AP view). Axial images are viewed as if we are viewing the patient from the feet, and the right of the image is the left of the patient and vice versa. On Figure B.7, all of the vessels that are identified are the patient's right cerebral arteries.

The majority of vessels within the head are known as cerebral arteries. The vessels that provide blood supply to the anterior portion of the brain are known as the left anterior cerebral arteries (lACA) and right anterior cerebral arteries (rACA) (see arrows A and B on Figure B.7). The vessels that provide blood supply to the middle portion of the brain are known as the left anterior cerebral arteries (lMCA) and right middle cerebral arteries (rMCA) (arrow C on Figure B.7). The vessels that provide blood supply to the posterior portion of the brain are known as the right posterior cerebral (rPCA) (arrow F on Figure B.7) and left posterior cerebral arteries (lPCA) (arrow G on Figure B.7)

There are small branches that "connect" or "communicates" between vessels. The vessel that "communicates" between the right and left anterior cerebral arteries is known as the anterior communicating artery (ACOM) (arrow D on Figure B.7) The vessel that "communicates" between the anterior and posterior cerebral arteries is known as the posterior communicating artery (PCOM) (arrow E on Figure B.7).

114. b

The high flow velocity in the brain requires 3D MRA techniques. 3D time of flight is better for small vascular structures with high flow velocities, especially when used with magnetization transfer techniques.

115. a

With the slower peripheral flow in the neck, 2D techniques are recommended so that blood flow is not suppressed along with stationary tissues.

116. c

Saturation pulses can be applied inferior to the acquired images to suppress the signal from venous blood (flowing up from the feet) and allow better visualization of arterial blood (flowing down from the heart).

117. b

This is a pneumonic that can be used to remember the 12 cranial nerves:

1.	On	Olfactory
2.	Old	Optic
3.	Olympus	Occulomotor
4.	Towering	Trochear
5.	Tops	Trigeminal
6.	A	Abducens
7.	Fin	Facial
8.	And	Acoustic/vestibulocochlear
9.	German	Glossopharyngeal
10.	Viewed	Vagus
11.	A	Accessory
12.	Hopps	Hypoglossal

118. d

According to the package insert for contrast media in MRI, the standard dosage of gadolinium is 0.2 mL/kg (cc per kilogram of body weight). This is equal to 0.1 mmol/kg (0.1 m/mol/kg of gadolinium or 10 cc for a 100 lb patient). Since there are 2.2 pounds to the kilogram, the standard dosage is equal to approximately 0.1 cc/lb.

119. d

120. c

121. c

122. b

123. a

124. c

125. d

126. e

Venous drainage of the head occurs whereby blood flows superiorly through superficial drainage veins and into the superior sagittal sinus and inferior sagittal sinus (not shown on Figure B.8). The inferior sagittal sinus drains into the straight sinus. Blood flows from the superior sagittal sinus and straight sinus – which join to from the confluence of sinuses. From there, blood flows into the sigmoid sinus (sigmoid, from the Latin, means "S"). The sigmoid sinus is a curved vessel. From the sigmoid sinus, blood flows into the internal jugular vein and then into the superior vena cava. Blood enters the heart by way of the superior and inferior vena cava.

127. a

128. a

129. a

130. b

131. c

132. c

133. d

134. c

135. a

The vessels that supply blood to the head and neck arise from the aortic arch. These are known as the "great vessels". Deoxygenated blood flows from the jugular veins into the superior vena cava (SVC). Deoxyhemoglobin (within the SVC) enters the right atrium of the heart, then the right ventricle, and through the pulmonary arteries to the lungs to acquire oxygen. From there, oxygen-rich blood (oxyhemoglobin) re-enters the heart by way of the left atrium and then the left ventricle; it is then "pumped" out of the heart by way of the ascending aorta.

Three "great vessels" arise off of the aortic arch. Remembering these vessels is as easy as "**ABCs**":

A. Blood flows through the **a**scending aorta.

B. The first vessel that arises at the arch is known as the **b**rachiocephalic artery. This vessel provides blood supply to the right arm (brachio) by way of the right subclavian artery; and to the head (cephalic) by way of the right common carotid artery and vertebral artery. The common carotid arteries bifurcate into the internal carotid artery (supplies blood to the frontal, temporal, and parietal lobes of the brain) and external carotid artery (supplies blood to structures "external" to the brain, such as the neck, face, and scalp). The right vertebral artery supplies blood to the posterior aspect of the head (occipital lobe and cerebellum).

C. The second vessel that originates on the aortic arch is the left **c**ommon carotid artery. This bifurcates into the internal carotid artery (supplies blood to the frontal, temporal, and parietal lobes of the brain) and external carotid artery (supplies blood to structures "external" to the brain, such as the neck, face, and scalp).

S. The third vessel that originates on the aortic arch is the left **s**ubclavian artery. The left vertebral artery supplies blood to the posterior aspect of the head (occipital lobe and cerebellum).

136. b

137. e

Discussion for brain imaging by MRI

Typical protocols for the evaluation of the anatomy of the brain consist of sagittal T1WI, and axial slices are selected for T2-, FLAIR, and diffusion-weighted images. Common pathology evaluated by MRI is listed in Table B.1. In addition, there are sequences, weighting, and imaging planes that are performed as the standard of care for particular pathologic conditions.

Table B.1 Common brain pathology evaluated by MRI.

Pathologic condition	Imaging plane	Centering and landmark	mage contrast
Stroke	Axial	For entire brain even though the majority of strokes occur in the region of the lacunar branches of the MCA MCA travels through the lateral or Sylvian fissure	Diffusion imaging Perfusion imaging MRA of the head (COW) MRA of the neck (carotids)
Vascular lesions of the head, such as aneurysm		3D TOF (for smaller vessels) like intracranial vessels, COW	
Vascular lesions of the neck, such as stenosis		2D TOF (for long areas of coverage), like extracranial vessels, carotid arteries of the neck	
Venous lesions of the head, such as sagittal sinus thrombosis		PCMRA (for flow direction and flow velocity)	
Seizures	Coronal	Hippocampus (temporal lobes)	T2WI and FLAIR
Sensory Neural Hearing loss	Coronal and axial	IACs	T2WI, T1WI + Gd
Pituitary adenoma	Sagittal and coronal	PIT (sella turcica)	T2WI, T1WI + Gd
Arnold–Chiari malformation	Sagittal		Craniocervical junction (brain + spinal cord for syrinx), high-resolution imaging
Infection, infarction, inflammation, neoplasm (tumor)			T1WI + Gd

COW, circle of Willis; IAC, internal auditory canal; PIT, pituitary; PCMRA, phase contrast magnetic resonance angiography; MCA, middle cerebral artery.

138. a

139. c

Scar enhances almost immediately after injection of contrast agents and will appear hyperintense to disk. However, after approximately 20 minutes, the disk will also enhance.

140. a

141. c

142. d

143. b

144. a

The spinal cord generally ends at the level of T12 or L1, and the cauda equina extends inferior to the conus. However, the exact location will vary from patient to patient, and with patient age. For this reason, MR imaging of the thoracic or lumbar spine (sagittal or coronal imaging planes) can be used to evaluate the conus and cauda equina.

145. b

146. a

147. a

148. c

149. d

150. b

151. c

152. b

153. a

154. e

155. c

There is sometimes a tendency to forget that the dens or the odontoid is C2. So when we "count" vertebral levels, remember to begin with C2, then C3, C4, and so on. There is no vertebral body for the first cervical level; therefore, on a midline sagittal view of the C-spine, only the anterior arch and posterior arch of C1 are visualized.

156. d

In general, 3D imaging provides all of these possibilities. In the C-spine, high-resolution 3D enables the visualization of small nerve roots. Also, if 3D gradient echo images are acquired with short TR, short TE, and small flip angle, T2* images can be created. If the flip angle is increased and the gradient echo is acquired with "spoiled" techniques, T1 gradient echoes are acquired. Finally, 3D acquisitions can be reconstructed (or reformatted) in multiple imaging planes.

157. b

158. a

159. d

160. c

161. b

162. b

163. c

164. d

165. b

166. a

167. b

168. c

169. e

170. b

171. a

172. a

173. b

174. a

175. b

176. e

177. c

178. a

179. d

180. d

181. e

182. d

183. d

184. b

185. d
This image can be identified as a T2WI (acquired with a long TR and long TE) since the fluid within the spinal canal is bright.

186. b

187. e

188. c
This can be identified as the intervertebral disk (rather than the vertebral body) on this axial oblique image, since the signal intensity is darker (in the region of the disk) compared to the higher signal in the bony components (pedicles, lamina, spinous process).

189. d

190. d

191. d

192. e

193. b

194. c

Discussion for spine imaging by MRI

Typical protocols for the evaluation of the anatomy of the spine consist of sagittal T1WI and selected axial slices for T2-, T1WI, and diffusion-weighted images (as needed) (Figure B.58). Common pathology evaluated by MRI is listed in Table B.2. In addition, there are sequences, weighting, and imaging planes that are performed as the standard of care for a particular pathologic condition.

Table B.2   Common spine pathology evaluated by MRI.

Pathologic condition	Imaging plane	Centering and landmark	Image contrast
Herniated disk	Cspine axial (oblique)	At the level of the suspected herniation	C-spine T1WI and T2*WI (3D gradient echo)
	Lspine oblique axial	At the level of the suspected herniation	L-spine T1WI + Gd for postop lumbar disk
Tumor	Any spinal location	At the level of the lesion	T1WI + Gd with fat suppression
Infection, infarction, inflammation, neoplasm (tumor)			T1WI + Gd
Arnold–Chiari malformation	Sagittal	Cranio-cervical junction	T1 and T2 high-resolution imaging
Conus tumor (bowel and bladder dysfunction)	Sagittal	Thoraco-lumbar junction	T1 and T2 high-resolution imaging
Scoliosis	Coronal and oblique	Complete spine	
	Oblique (to create images axial and/or sagittal to the plane of the "curves" spinal canal)		
Brachial plexus	Coronal or sagittal	Nerves originate at the level of C4–T1. Coil position and patient centering, approximately at the clavicle	T1 and T1

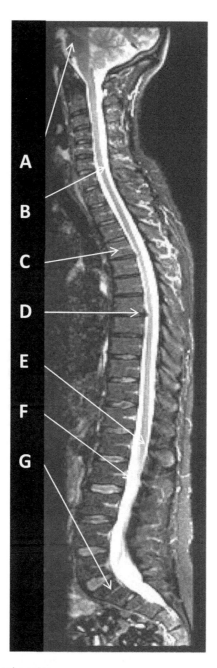

Figure B.58 MRI of spinal anatomy.

195. c

196. a

197. a

198. b

199. a

200. c

201. d

202. c

203. a

204. e

Discussion for thorax imaging by MRI

The visualization of MR images is the same as the visualization of radiographic images, whereby we "face" the anatomic man (the patient). As a result, the right side of the image is the left of the patient. In Figure B.10, a coronal T1-weighted image of the thorax, the patient is facing us. For this reason, the right side of the image is the left of the patient (and vice-versa). The heart is located primarily within the left of the thorax. For this reason, the heart occupies a considerable amount of space within the midline (mediastinum) of the thorax. The lungs consist of several lobes. The right lung consists of three lobes [right superior lobe (or apex of the lung), the right middle lobe and the right inferior lobe (or the base of the lung)]. Since the heart occupies space within the left thorax, the left lung consists of two lobes [left superior lobe (or apex) and the inferior lobe (or base)].

205. c

206. a

207. d

208. b

Discussion for cardiac gating or triggering

Motion artifact is most likely the leading cause of the degradation of image quality in MRI. Imaging the thorax poses many challenges as structures within the chest are associated with motion in the "living" patient. Motion can be divided into several categories, including periodic and aperiodic motion. The effects of periodic motion can be corrected (or compensated) more easily than aperiodic motion effects. For chest imaging, both periodic and aperiodic motion should be considered. Types of physiologic motion, and compensation techniques for them, include:

Periodic motion

1. Cardiac motion
   - The "beating" heart causes pulsatile (periodic) motion
   - Scanning can be timed (triggered or gated) to the heart beat. Triggering or gating can be performed:
     ○ Prospectively (Figure B.59) – the scan is "timed" to the heart beat. The scan is acquired at appropriate "times" during the cardiac cycle:
       – With prospective gating, the scan is "initiated" by the R-wave
       – There is a user selectable parameter known as the % trigger window that is selected to allow for the R-wave to be initiated:
       If the heart rate is 60 bpm, the R–R interval is 1000 ms
       10% delay after trigger – "uses" 100 ms
       – The delay after trigger is a user-selectable parameter that allows for the specific time that imaging begins (during systole or diastole):
       If a 50 ms delay is selected, another 50 ms is "used"
       – The available imaging time (AIT) is the time during which slices can be acquired:
       Begin with 1000 ms, subtract 100 ms (% window) and subtract 50 ms (delay)
       In this example, the AIT is 850 ms (AIT = time permitted to acquire slices)
     ○ Retrospectively (Figure B.60) – the scan is acquired throughout the cardiac cycle and "sorted" later (during image reconstruction):
       – With retrospective gating, scanning is performed throughout the cardiac cycle
       – How many images can be acquired during the cardiac cycle?
       If the R–R interval is 1000 ms
       If the TR is 25 ms
       1000 ms divided by 25 ms TR = 40 phases of the cardiac cycle

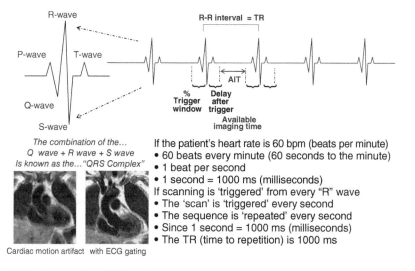

The combination of the...
Q wave + R wave + S wave
Is known as the..."QRS Complex"

Cardiac motion artifact with ECG gating

If the patient's heart rate is 60 bpm (beats per minute)
- 60 beats every minute (60 seconds to the minute)
- 1 beat per second
- 1 second = 1000 ms (milliseconds)
If scanning is 'triggered' from every "R" wave
- The 'scan' is 'triggered' every second
- The sequence is 'repeated' every second
- Since 1 second = 1000 ms (milliseconds)
- The TR (time to repetition) is 1000 ms

Figure B.59 Prospective ECG gating (or cardiac triggering)

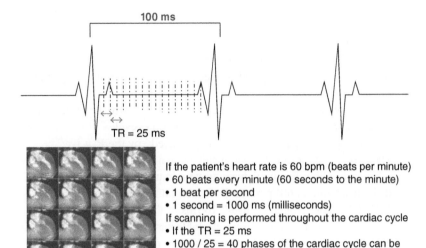

If the patient's heart rate is 60 bpm (beats per minute)
• 60 beats every minute (60 seconds to the minute)
• 1 beat per second
• 1 second = 1000 ms (milliseconds)
If scanning is performed throughout the cardiac cycle
• If the TR = 25 ms
• 1000 / 25 = 40 phases of the cardiac cycle can be imaged

Cardiac cine acquisition with 16 phases

Figure B.60   Retrospective cardiac gating.

2. Arteries and veins
- "The great vessels" within the chest. Arterial flood (and also to a certain extent venous flow) cause pulsatile flow motion

3. The diaphragm and lungs (cause respiratory motion)

Aperiodic motion

1. Patient motion

2. Swallowing associated with the esophagus (during swallowing)

3. Peristalsis associated with the stomach (gastric motion during digestion)

209. a

210. d

MR imaging is typically performed for the evaluation of "soft tissue" structures within the body. The image in Figure B.15 has been acquired with short TR, short TE, and small flip angle gradient echo (T2*). These selections will produce a gradient echo acquisition whereby flowing blood is bright.

Spin echo acquisitions can be acquired with T1, T2, or PD contrast. Gradient echo images can also be acquired with T1, T2*, or PD image contrast. On spin echo images, flowing blood is dark. On gradient echo acquisitions, flowing blood is bright. The image in Figure B.19 has high signal for flowing blood within the vessels in the lungs and within the heart.

211. d

212. c

213. b

214. a

215. e

216. f

217. d

218. b

219. a

220. c

221. a

222. e

223. d

224. c

225. d

226. b

227. c

228. c

229. a

230. d

231. d

232. d

233. c

234. b

235. d

236. e

237. e

238. d

239. a

240. b

241. d

242. b

243. c

244. b

245. c

246. d

247. e

248. a

249. b

250. c

Discussion for cardiac imaging by MRI

Blood flow enters the heart by way of the superior vena cava (SVC) and the inferior vena cava (IVC). Deoxyhemoglobin (within the SVC and IVC) enters the right atrium (RA) of the heart. From the RA, blood flows through the tricuspid valve into the right ventricle (RV). The RV is the most anterior chamber of the heart, located just behind the sternum. Blood from the RV travels through the pulmonary semilunar valve and into the pulmonary arteries. Note:

- All arteries carry oxyhemoglobin (oxygenated or oxygen-rich blood) away from the heart and to a structure, EXCEPT the pulmonary arteries (PA).
- The PA carry blood away from the heart and to a structure (the lungs) BUT this blood is deoxygenated (i.e. carrying deoxyhemoglobin).

Pulmonary arteries carry deoxyhemoglobin (deoxygenated or oxygen poor blood) into the capillaries around the alveoli to obtain oxygen (O_2) from the lungs and deposit carbon dioxide (CO_2). Next, blood flows into venules and then the pulmonary veins to be returned to the heart. Note:

- All veins carry deoxyhemoglobin (deoxygenated or oxygen-poor blood) away from a structure and to the heart, EXCEPT the pulmonary veins (PV).
- The PV carry blood to the heart and away from a structure (the lungs), but carry oxy-hemoglobin (oxygenated or oxygen-rich blood.).
- Another exception to this "rule" is the portal vein. The portal vein carries deoxyhemo-globin (deoxygenated or oxygen-poor blood) like other veins; however, this blood travels to the liver.

From the PV, oxygen-rich blood enters the heart via the left atrium (LA). The LA is the most posterior chamber of the heart and is located just anterior to the thoracic spine. From the LA, blood flows through the bicuspid (or mitral) valve. (When it comes to "heart valves", remember to *tri* before you *bi* – the tricuspid valve is between the atrium and ventricle of the right heart and tricuspid, the left.) From the tricuspid (or mitral) valve, blood flows into the left ventricle (LV). The LV pumps blood out of the heart and into the aorta (to supply blood to the entire body). Since the LV has a great task (of supplying blood to the entire body), the chamber of the heart with the "thickest" wall muscle (myocardium) is the left ventricle. Blood "leaves" the heart by way of the aortic valve and flows into the ascending aorta. The heart "feeds" itself first – the first "branches" that arise from the ascending aorta are the coronary arteries. The right coronaries "feed" the right heart and the left coronaries "feed" the left heart. The aorta ascends superiorly and forms an "arch". Three branches that arise from the arch, known as the great vessels. These vessels supply blood to the upper part of the body, including the arms, neck, and head. The blood flows through the aorta, continues around the arch, inferiorly through the thoracic aorta, and then down to the abdominal aorta.

MR imaging can be performed for the evaluation of the heart. This imaging can be challenging as the heart is "oblique" to the plane of the thorax. For this reason, multiple oblique views are required. To acquire the short axis view (axial to the plane of the heart muscle), images can be acquired perpendicular to the line from the apex of the heart to the base of the heart. Once the short axis view is acquired, two-chamber (long axis or sagittal to the heart) or long axis (sagittal to the heart) views can be acquired. For long axis views, images are acquired parallel to the interventricular septum. For four- chamber views, images are acquired perpendicular to the interventricular septum. View the images in Figure B.18.

For the evaluation of a patient with myocardial infarction (MI), commonly known as a heart attack, dynamic contrast-enhanced perfusion imaging is performed. Imaging is typically performed with T1 gradient echo acquisitions before and several "passes" after contrast enhancement. The short axis view of the left ventricle is the most common view for the evaluation of patients with MI.

251. a

252. c

253. b

254. d

255. b

256. d

257. a

258. a

259. b

260. c

261. d

262. e

Discussion for spin echo and gradient echo imaging by MRI

MR imaging can be performed with either spin echo (SE) or gradient echo (GrE) acquisitions. Typically SE sequences provide higher quality but longer scan times, and GrE sequences provide lower image quality but faster scan times. Also, GrE sequences have typical characteristics and artifacts, including high signal from flowing blood, susceptibility artifact (from metal, blood, and differences in tissue types), and chemical shift artifact (where fat and water interface). These effects and artifacts are demonstrated in Figure B.19.

263. a

264. b

265. b

266. c

267. f

268. d

269. d

270. a

271. e

272. d

273. e

274. b

275. a

276. d

277. b

278. f

279. d

280. c

281. d

282. b

283. c

Discussion for breast MRI

Breast lesions

MR imaging of the breast (for the evaluation of breast lesions) is typically performed with high-resolution imaging protocols and with T1, T2, and gradient echo T1 fat-suppressed dynamic contrast enhancement. Such protocols include either high-resolution, unilateral (or bilateral) sagittal imaging (the so-called US method) or high-resolution axial bilateral imaging (the so-called European method or Porter method). The American College of Radiology (ACR) recommends that high-resolution imaging is performed with 1-mm in-plane resolution, whereby pixel size is 1 mm. The high-resolution recommendation also includes 3–4-mm through-plane resolution, whereby slice thickness is 3 or 4 mm.

Silicone implants

Silicone breast implants are constructed of a polyurethane (plastic) bag filled with a "sticky" substance (silicone). In the event that the polyurethane (plastic) bag ruptures, silicone can "leak" out of the "bag" and migrate through the body. When implants are surgically "placed" within the body, a scar-like tissue, known as the "capsule" forms around the surgical site.

MR imaging of the breast for the evaluation of silicone breast implants is typically performed with high-resolution imaging protocols (sagittal or bilateral axial) with suppression techniques. This allows for the visualization of the breast, the implant, and the potential "rupture" of the implant. Such protocols include either high-resolution sagittal imaging or high-resolution axial imaging. Imaging is performed to determine if the silicone implant has ruptured or remains intact. Suppression techniques can be performed for the suppression of fat (fat sat and/or STIR), water suppression (water sat and/or FLAIR), or silicone suppression. To acquire images whereby the silicone is bright and other structures darker, STIR is used to suppress fat and water sat is used to suppress water. In Figure B.61 silicone remains bright. If, however imaging is to be performed

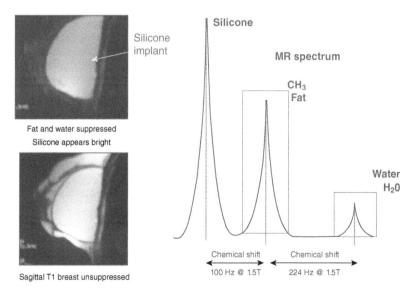

Figure B.61 Breast implants: fat and water suppression.

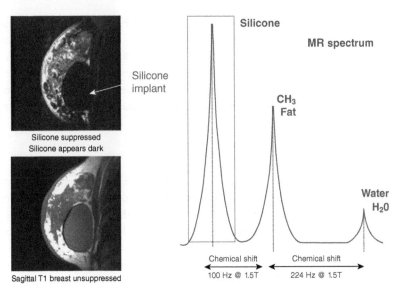

Figure B.62 Breast implants: silicone suppression.

Table B.3 Common breast pathology evaluated by MRI.

Pathologic condition	Imaging plane	Centering and landmark	Image contrast
Breast MR for lesions	Axial, high resolution	Breasts to isocenter	T1, T2, and T1 GrE with dynamic Gd Enhancement with fat suppression
	Sagittal, high resolution	Breasts to isocenter	T1, T2, and T1 GrE with dynamic Gd Enhancement with fat suppression
Breast MR for implants	Sagittal or axial	Breasts to isocenter	Fat and water suppression, or silicone suppression

whereby the silicone is dark and other structures brighter, silicone suppression is used to suppress silicone (Figure B.62).

Once the breast is imaged and it is confirmed that the implant has ruptured, it is important to determine if the silicone is within the 'capsule' (intra-capsular rupture) or has leaked out of the 'capsule' (extra-capsular rupture).

Common pathology evaluated by MRI is listed in Table B.3.

284. c

285. b

286. e

287. d

288. c

289. b

290. e

291. a

292. a

293. a

294. c

295. b

296. d

297. b

Discussion for abdominal motion/artifact

Motion artifact is most likely the leading cause for the degradation of image quality in MRI. Imaging the abdomen poses many challenges as structures within the torso are associated with motion in the "living" patient. Motion can be divided into several categories, including periodic and aperiodic motion. The effects of periodic motion can be corrected (or compensated) more easily than aperiodic motion effects. For abdomen imaging, both periodic and aperiodic motion should be considered. Types of physiologic motion, and compensation techniques for them, include:

Periodic motion

1. Respiratory motion and respiratory gating or triggering (Figure B.63)
   - The respiratory cycle creates (periodic) motion
   - Scanning can be timed (triggered or gated) to the respiratory cycle. Triggering or gating can be performed by monitoring the respiratory rate and scanning either prospectively or retrospectively:
     - Prospectively – the scan is "timed" to the respiratory beat. The scan is acquired at appropriate "times" during the respiratory cycle'. If the normal respiratory rate is 12 breaths per minute, then (as there are 60 seconds per minute) scan timing would be approximately every 4–5 seconds. In this case the TR would be 4000 or 5000 ms.
     - Retrospectively – this technique is known as ROPE (respiratory ordered phase encoding). The scans acquired throughout the respiratory cycle and phase encoding steps are "sorted" later (during image reconstruction)

Aperiodic abdominal motion

1. Patient motion
2. Peristalsis associated with the stomach (gastric motion during digestion)

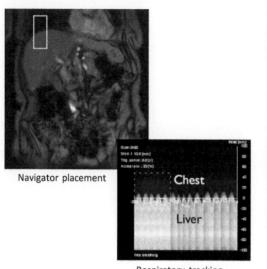

Navigator placement

Respiratory tracking

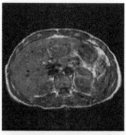

Respiratory motion artifact

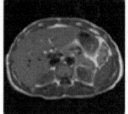

With respiratory triggering

Figure B.63   Respiratory triggering.

298. a

299. a

300. a

301. b

302. d

303. c

304. a

305. b

306. c

307. d

308. e

309. d

310. a

311. a

312. b

313. c

314. a

315. d

316. b

317. c

318. a

319. c

320. b

321. d

322. a

323. c

324. d

325. f

326. b

327. d

328. c

329. b

330. c

331. d

332. a

333. b

334. c

335. d

336. c

337. a

338. b

339. d

340. d

341. e

342. d

Timing for enhanced liver imaging is essential as many cancerous liver lesions are visualized on the first pass. To identify the phases of enhancement, one must understand that the first (arterial) phase demonstrates the following:

- Spleen is hyperintense to (brighter than) liver
- Spleen shows "mottled" or "marbled" enhancement
- Only the cortex of the kidneys are enhanced

343. a

344. c

Since most liver cancers are "arterially fed", they are best visualized on the first pass. In contrast, other lesions (hemangiomas) are demonstrated with delayed enhancement.

345. a

346. a

347. b

348. a

349. d

350. d

351. b

352. d

353. d

354. c

355. c

356. c

357. e

358. a

359. c

360. b

361. c

362. d

363. b

364. e

365. e

366. b

367. a

368. b

369. b

370. d

371. d

372. b

373. a

374. c

375. b

376. c

377. d

378. a

379. b

380. d

381. e

382. b

383. c

384. a

385. d

386. d

387. d

388. e

389. a

390. c

391. d

392. d

393. e

394. d

395. c

396. d

397. b

398. c

399. d

400. a

401. b

402. c

403. d

404. d

405. d

406. e

407. d

408. a

409. c

410. a

411. b

412. a

413. b

414. c

415. c

416. d

417. c

418. c

419. a

420. b

421. a

422. d

423. c

424. e

425. d

426. a

427. d

428. b

429. b

430. c

431. b

432. e

433. a

434. d

435. a

436. c

437. c

438. d

439. d

440. b

441. a

442. a

443. c

444. c
When evaluating the musculoskeletal system for "range of motion", images are acquired during movement of the joint. This technique is known as kinematic imaging or musculoskeletal ciné. Figure B.38 demonstrates images with the mouth closed (top) and opened (bottom). When the mouth is opened, the condyle moves forward out of the temporal bone groove. The images to the right have a normal meniscus, while the images to the left have a torn meniscus.

445. a

446. b

447. a

448. c

449. d

450. c

451. d

452. a

453. b

454. c

455. c

456. c
Tendons extend from muscle to bone. Ligaments extend from bone to bone. The structures that make up the rotator cuff include "SITS": **S**upraspinatus muscle and

tendon, **I**nfraspinatus muscle and tendon, **T**eres minor muscle and tendon, and **S**ubscapularis muscle and tendon. These tendons extend to (and attach to) the lateral aspect of the humeral head.

457. b

458. b

459. b

460. e

461. a

462. c

463. b

464. a

465. b

466. c

467. d

468. d

469. d

470. a

471. b

472. c

473. d

474. b

475. b

476. a

477. c

478. a

479. b

480. a

481. a

482. a

483. b

484. d

485. e

486. c

487. d

488. d

489. a

490. d

491. b

Remember that the olecraonon process is visualized like the "sunrise" view of the knee (patella). Remember also that when we view images, we view them as if we were facing the "anatomic man". The anatomic man is flat footed, and facing forward with palms facing forward. In this case, the olecranon process would be located posterior.

492. b

493. e

494. c

495. c

496. a

497. d

498. d

499. a

500. c

501. b

502. e

503. b

504. c

505. b

506. a

507. b

508. c

509. d

510. c

511. a

512. b

513. c

514. d

515. c

516. b

517. d

518. c

519. c

520. b

521. a

522. b

523. a

524. b

525. b

526. a

527. b

528. c

529. e

530. d

531. a

532. c

533. b

534. c

535. a

536. c

537. d

538. b

539. a

540. b

541. d

542. b

543. a

544. a

545. b

546. c

547. a

548. b

549. e

550. d

551. c

552. d

553. c

554. a

555. c

556. a

557. a

558. b

559. a

560. b

561. a

562. c

563. d

564. a

565. f

566. a

567. c

568. a

569. d

570. a

571. d

572. a

573. e

574. b

575. b

576. a

577. a

578. a

579. b

580. c

581. d

582. b

583. c

584. d

585. b

586. c

587. a

588. b

589. c

590. b

591. a

592. d

593. e

594. a

Part C

Data Acquisition and Processing

Image Parameters, Pulse Sequences, Spatial Localization, and Image Quality

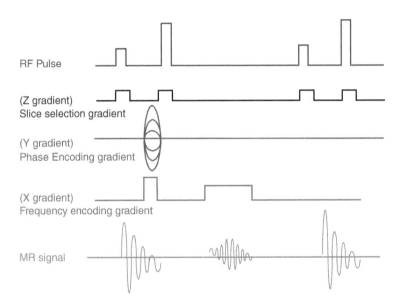

Introduction

MR images can be thought of as having three major components: contrast, signal-to-noise ratio (SNR), and spatial resolution. Many MR parameters that are under operator control can determine image contrast, SNR, and spatial resolution. In addition, tissue characteristics such as individual molecular make-up, disease state, and field strength influence image contrast, SNR, and resolution.

Review Questions for MRI, Second Edition. Carolyn Kaut Roth and William H. Faulkner.
© 2013 Carolyn Kaut Roth and William S. Faulkner. Published 2013 by Blackwell Publishing Ltd.

The extrinsic, or operator-controlled, parameters that affect an image's contrast, SNR, and spatial resolution are interrelated. The type of acquisition used (i.e. 2D or 3D Fourier transform) can also affect the contrast and SNR of the images, and is often a critical consideration in developing protocols or deciding what type of sequence to perform. Additionally, the sequence selected may produce images in which some amount of image or data processing is required. It is critical for the technologist to understand these inter-relationships between parameters, and to know how to manipulate the user-selectable parameters to produce images suitable for interpretation.

Part C offers review questions that pertain to data acquisition and processing.

Type of study	Focus of questions

1. Pulse sequences
  a. Spin echo
    • Conventional spin echo
    • Fast spin echo (FSE)
  b. Inversion recovery
    • STIR
    • FLAIR
  c. Gradient recall echo (GRE)
    • Conventional gradient echo
    • Fast gradient echo
  d. Echo planar imaging (EPI)
  e. Calibration scans
    • Filtering
    • Parallel imaging
2. Data manipulation
  a. K-space mapping and filling
  b. Fourier transformation
  c. Post processing
    • Maximum intensity projection (MIP)
    • Multiplanar reconstruction techniques (MPR)
    • Subtraction
    • Volume rendering
  d. Cardiac analysis
3. Special procedures
  a. MRA/MRV
    • Flow dynamics
    • Time-of-flight
    • Phase contrast
    • Contrast enhanced
    • Fluoro-triggering
    • Timing bolus
    • Automatic bolus detection (e.g. smart prep, care bolus)
  b. Functional techniques
    • Diffusion
    • Perfusion
    • Spectroscopy
    • fMRI
  c. Dynamic imaging
	Questions will address the interdependence of the imaging parameters and options listed on the left, and how those parameters and options affect image quality and contrast.
	1. Image quality
	  • Contrast to noise (C/N)
	  • Signal to noise (S/N)
	  • Spatial resolution
	  • Acquisition time
	2. Contrast
	  • T1 weighted
	  • T2 weighted
	  • proton (spin) density
	  • T2* weighted

Type of study	Focus of questions

4. Sequence parameters and options
  a. Imaging parameters
    • TR
    • TE
    • TI
    • Number of signal averages (NSA)
    • Flip angle (Ernst angle)
    • FOV
    • Matrix
    • Number of slices
    • Slice thickness and gap
    • Phase and frequency
    • Echo train length
    • Effective TE
  b. Imaging options
    • 2D/3D
    • Bandwidth
    • Slice order
    • Saturation pulse
    • Gradient moment nulling
    • Suppression techniques (e.g. fat, water, etc.)
    • Selective excitation
    • Physiologic gating and triggering
    • In-phase/out-of-phase
    • Rectangular FOV
    • Anti-aliasing
    • Parallel imaging	

Questions 1–63 concern pulse sequences, questions 64–88 data manipulation, questions 89–125 special procedures, and questions 126–193 sequence parameters and options.

Part C: Questions

Pulse sequences

1. An inversion recovery (IR) spin echo sequence begins with a:

> **a.** 90° RF pulse ☐
> **b.** 180° RF pulse ☐
> **c.** 45° RF pulse ☐
> **d.** a or b ☐

2. A typical spin echo (SE) sequence uses pulses:

> **a.** 90°, 90° ☐
> **b.** 90°, 180° ☐
> **c.** 180°, 180° ☐
> **d.** 180°, 90° ☐

3. A typical inversion recovery (IR) spin echo sequence uses pulses:

> **a.** 90°, 180°, 180° ☐
> **b.** 180°, 90°, 180° ☐
> **c.** 5° RF pulse ☐
> **d.** a or b ☐

4. T2-weighted fluid attenuated inversion recovery (FLAIR) sequences are typically used for the evaluation of:

> **a.** Musculoskeletal contusions ☐
> **b.** Fat ☐
> **c.** Retro-orbital fat ☐
> **d.** Periventricular white matter disease ☐

5. A typical gradient echo sequence begins with a:

> **a.** 90° RF pulse ☐
> **b.** 180° RF pulse ☐
> **c.** Alpha pulse that varies with desired image contrast ☐
> **d.** Alpha pulse below 10° ☐

6. Short tau inversion recovery (STIR) sequences are typically used for the evaluation of all of the following EXCEPT:

a. Musculoskeletal contusions ☐
b. Fat suppression ☐
c. Lesions within the retro-orbital fat ☐
d. Fluid (CSF) ☐

7. STIR sequences can suppress the signal from all of the following EXCEPT:

a. Fat within bone marrow ☐
b. Gadolinium-enhancing lesions ☐
c. Retro-orbital fat ☐
d. Fluid (CSF) ☐

8. To produce the echo, a gradient echo pulse sequence uses a:

a. Gradient magnetic field only ☐
b. RF pulse only ☐
c. Combination of a and b ☐
c. Switching device ☐
d. A combination of any two RF pulses ☐

9. The 180° pulse that follows the initial 90° pulse in a spin echo sequence will cause the NMR signal to reappear while correcting for:

a. Slight magnetic field inhomogeneities ☐
b. Chemical shift ☐
c. Slight magnetic susceptibility effects ☐
d. All of the above ☐

10. The gradient that is on during the production of the echo is called the:

a. Phase encoding gradient ☐
b. Slice select gradient ☐
c. Frequency encoding gradient/readout gradient ☐
d. Flow encoding gradient ☐

11. If the TR of a gradient echo pulse sequence is considerably less than the T2 (and T2*), the condition that will exist is known as:

    a. Steady state ☐
    b. Spin dephasing ☐
    c. Spin rephrasing ☐
    d. Spin cancellation ☐

12. Phase encoding is performed:

    a. After frequency encoding ☐
    b. Prior to frequency encoding ☐
    c. In place of frequency encoding ☐
    d. During frequency encoding ☐

13. The gradient that is on during the production of the echo is the:

    a. Phase ☐
    b. Slice selection ☐
    c. Frequency ☐
    d. Oblique ☐

14. The "readout" gradient is also known as the:

    a. Phase ☐
    b. Slice selection ☐
    c. Frequency ☐
    d. Oblique ☐

15. If a phase resolution of 256 is desired, then the TR must be repeated (for one NSA):

    a. 192 times ☐
    b. 256 times ☐
    c. 512 times ☐
    d. Twice ☐

16. In the multi-echo spin echo sequence shown in Figure C.1, the number of SHORT TE images created with a 20-slice sequence will be:

    a. 2 ☐
    b. 4 ☐
    c. 20 ☐
    d. 40 ☐

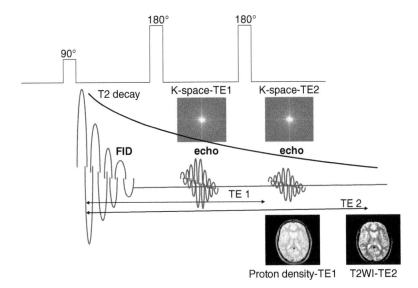

Figure C.1

17. In the multi-echo spin echo sequence shown in Figure C.1, the number of LONG TE images created with a 20-slice sequence will be:

a. 2 ☐
b. 4 ☐
c. 20 ☐
d. 40 ☐

18. In the multi-echo spin echo sequence shown in Figure C.1, the number of images PER SLICE LOCATION created will be:

a. 2 ☐
b. 4 ☐
c. 20 ☐
d. 40 ☐

19. In the multi-echo spin echo sequence shown in Figure C.1, the TOTAL number of images created with a 20-slice sequence will be:

a. 2 ☐
b. 4 ☐
c. 20 ☐
d. 40 ☐

20. In the multi-echo spin echo sequence shown in Figure C.1, images will be acquired with varying amounts of:

a. T1 information ☐
b. T2 information ☐
c. T2* information ☐
d. Proton density (PD) information ☐

21. If the pulse sequence shown in Figure C.1 were a fast spin echo sequence, the number of lines of K space filled during each TR period would be:

a. 4 ☐
b. 1 ☐
c. 8 ☐
d. 2 ☐

22. If a given conventional spin echo pulse sequence takes 12 minutes to acquire, a fast spin echo sequence using an ETL of six, with all other factors that affect scan time remaining the same, will take:

a. 2 minutes ☐
b. 1 minute ☐
c. 6 minutes ☐
d. 4 minutes ☐

23. In a fast spin echo sequence, the effective TE is the echo that is performed with the:

a. Outer views of K space ☐
b. High amplitude phase-encoding gradients ☐
c. Low amplitude phase-encoding gradients ☐
d. First phase-encoding steps ☐

24. In a fast spin echo sequence, spatial resolution is associated with the:

a. Central lines of K space ☐
b. High amplitude phase-encoding gradients ☐
c. Low amplitude phase-encoding gradients ☐
d. First phase-encoding steps ☐

25. In a fast spin echo (FSE) sequence, acquired with short effective TE (T1- or PD-weighted images), blurring can be reduced by the selection of:

- **a.** Shorter ETL ☐
- **b.** Longer ETL ☐
- **c.** There is no ETL change that affects blurring ☐
- **d.** Larger FOV ☐

26. In a fast spin echo (FSE) sequence, acquired with long effective TE (T2-weighted images), scan time can be reduced by the selection of:

- **a.** Shorter ETL ☐
- **b.** Longer ETL ☐
- **c.** There is no ETL change that affects scan time ☐
- **d.** Larger FOV ☐

27. A gradient echo sequence in which any residual transverse magnetization is removed prior to the next excitation pulse is known as:

- **a.** Nonphasic ☐
- **b.** Incoherent/spoiled ☐
- **c.** Nonresidual ☐
- **d.** Magnetization prepared ☐

28. When a gradient echo sequence is acquired for dynamic contrast-enhanced imaging of the liver, _____ is performed.

- **a.** An additional 180° pulse ☐
- **b.** An initial 180° pulse ☐
- **c.** Spoiling ☐
- **d.** Coherence ☐

29. Gradient echo sequences acquired for high signal from fluid are known as all of the following EXCEPT:

- **a.** Coherent gradient echoes ☐
- **b.** Incoherent gradient echoes ☐
- **c.** Steady-state gradient echoes ☐
- **d.** T2* gradient echoes ☐

30. Dynamic enhanced MRA sequences of the renal arteries are performed with the use of:

> **a.** Incoherent gradient echoes ☐
> **b.** Coherent gradient echoes ☐
> **c.** Steady-state gradient echoes ☐
> **d.** T2* gradient echoes ☐

31. Gradient echo sequences can yield either T1 or T2* characteristics.

> **a.** True ☐
> **b.** False ☐

32. Gradient echo sequences can yield either T1 or T2* characteristics, with influences caused by all of the following EXCEPT:

> **a.** Susceptibility ☐
> **b.** Inhomogeneity ☐
> **c.** Chemical shift ☐
> **d.** Aliasing ☐

33. Gradient echo sequences acquired for the evaluation of hemorrhagic lesions rely on:

> **a.** Susceptibility ☐
> **b.** Inhomogeneity ☐
> **c.** Chemical shift ☐
> **d.** Aliasing ☐

34. A FLAIR sequence is utilized to suppress the signal from:

> **a.** MS plaques ☐
> **b.** Gadolinium ☐
> **c.** Fat ☐
> **d.** CSF ☐

35. Which of the following field strengths would require the shortest (lowest) TI time to suppress/null the signal from fat when acquiring a STIR sequence in an MR exam of the knee?

> **a.** 0.35 T ☐
> **b.** 1.0 T ☐
> **c.** 1.5 T ☐
> **d.** 3.0 T ☐

36. If one desires to null the signal from a specific tissue using an inversion recovery sequence, one should select an inversion time that is _____ of the T1 relaxation time of that tissue.

a. 43% ☐
b. 69% ☐
c. 80% ☐
d. 37% ☐

37. Which of the following best describes an EPI sequence?

a. A 90° pulse followed by a 180° pulse ☐
b. A 180° pulse followed by a 90°/180° combination ☐
c. A "train" of gradient echoes ☐
d. A "train" of spin echoes ☐

38. Which of the following best describes an FSE sequence?

a. A 90° pulse followed by a 180° pulse ☐
b. A 180° pulse followed by a 90°/180° combination ☐
c. A "train" of gradient echoes ☐
d. A "train" of spin echoes ☐

39. Which of the following best describes an IR sequence?

a. A 90° pulse followed by a 180° pulse ☐
b. A 180° pulse followed by a 90°/180° combination ☐
c. A "train" of gradient echoes ☐
d. A "train" of spin echoes ☐

40. Which of the following best describes a SE sequence?

a. A 90° pulse followed by a 180° pulse ☐
b. A 180° pulse followed by a 90°/180° combination ☐
c. A "train" of gradient echoes ☐
d. A "train" of spin echoes ☐

41. In which of the following EPI sequences would one expect there to be the least susceptibility (distortion) artifacts?

a. Single-shot SE-EPI, 256 phase × 256 frequency ☐
b. Single-shot GRE-EPI, 512 phase × 192 frequency ☐
c. Multi-shot (4-shot) SE-EPI, 256 phase × 256 frequency ☐
d. Single-shot SE-EPI, 192 phase × 192 frequency ☐

42. When acquiring an fMRI series to map out the visual cortex, which of the following pulse sequences would be utilized in order to maximize sensitivity to the BOLD effect?

> **a.** Spin echo EPI ☐
> **b.** Gradient echo EPI ☐
> **c.** Fast spin echo with driven equilibrium ☐
> **d.** 3D spoiled GRE with MTC ☐

43. In which of the following sequences would MS plaques appear hyperintense relative to both CSF and normal white matter?

> **a.** T2 FLAIR ☐
> **b.** T1 FLAIR ☐
> **c.** T2 FSE ☐
> **d.** T2 FSE with RF fat suppression ☐

44. In a balanced GRE acquisition, the contrast weighting is:

> **a.** T1 weighted ☐
> **b.** T2 weighted ☐
> **c.** T2* weighted ☐
> **d.** Weighted for the ratio of T2/T1 ☐

45. In an image acquired with a balanced GRE sequence (Figure C.2), all of the following have high (bright) signal EXCEPT:

> **a.** Blood in the left ventricle ☐
> **b.** CSF ☐
> **c.** IVC ☐
> **d.** Normal myocardium ☐

46. Parallel imaging techniques are also known as all of the following EXCEPT:

> **a.** SENSE ☐
> **b.** SMASH ☐
> **c.** GRAPPA ☐
> **d.** SAT ☐

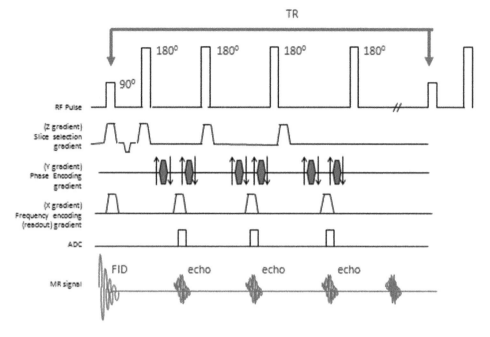

Figure C.2

47. When parallel imaging techniques are performed, a low resolution _____ scan is acquired prior to the acquisition:

    a. Test bolus ☐
    b. Filtering scan ☐
    c. Calibration scan ☐
    d. Sat pulse ☐

48. When doing an MRA of the IVC, a saturation band should be placed _____ to the axial slices.

    a. Anterior ☐
    b. Posterior ☐
    c. Superior ☐
    d. Inferior ☐

49. When doing an MRA of the carotid arteries, a saturation band should be placed _____ to the axial slices.

    a. Anterior ☐
    b. Posterior ☐
    c. Superior ☐
    d. Inferior ☐

50. When doing an MRA of the circle of Willis, a saturation band should be placed _____ to the axial slices.

    a. Anterior ☐
    b. Posterior ☐
    c. Superior ☐
    d. Inferior ☐

51. When doing an MRV of the superior sagittal sinus, a saturation band should be placed _____ to the axial slices.

    a. Anterior ☐
    b. Posterior ☐
    c. Superior ☐
    d. Inferior ☐

52. Scan time for 2D SE pulse sequences can be calculated by:

    a. $TR \times \#PEs \times NSA$ ☐
    b. $TR \times \#PEs \times NSA \times \#slices$ ☐
    c. $TR \times \#PEs \times NSA/ETL$ ☐
    d. $TR \times \#shots \times NSA$ ☐

53. Scan time for 2D IR pulse sequences can be calculated by:

    a. $TR \times \#PEs \times NSA$ ☐
    b. $TR \times \#PEs \times NSA \times \#slices$ ☐
    c. $TR \times \#PE's \times NSA/ETL$ ☐
    d. $TR \times \#shots \times NSA$ ☐

54. Scan time for 2D GRE pulse sequences can be calculated by:

    a. $TR \times \#PEs \times NSA$ ☐
    b. $TR \times \#PEs \times NSA \times \# slices$ ☐
    c. $TR \times \#PEs \times NSA/ETL$ ☐
    d. $TR \times \#shots \times NSA$ ☐

55. Scan time for EPI pulse sequences can be calculated by:

    a. $TR \times \#PEs \times NSA$ ☐
    b. $TR \times \#PEs \times NSA \times \#slices$ ☐
    c. $TR \times \#PEs \times NSA \times ETL$ ☐
    d. $TR \times \#shots \times NSA$ ☐

56. Scan time for 2D FSE pulse sequences can be calculated by:

a. TR × #PEs × NSA ☐
b. TR × #PEs × NSA × #slices ☐
c. TR × #PEs s NSA/ETL ☐
d. TR × #shots × NSA ☐

57. Scan time for a "volume" acquisition can be calculated by:

a. TR × #PEs × NSA ☐
b. TR × #PEs × NSA × #slices ☐
c. TR × #PEs × NSA/ETL ☐
d. TR × #shots × NSA ☐

58. In a fast spin echo pulse sequence, if the echo trail length is increased by a factor of four, the scan will be:

a. One times as fast ☐
b. Twice as fast ☐
c. Three times as fast ☐
d. Four times as fast ☐

59. In a volume acquisition, the scan time is:

a. TR × NSA × BW × thickness ☐
b. TR × NSA × phase encodings × slab thickness ☐
c. TR × NSA × number of phase encodings × ETL ☐
d. TR × NSA × number of phase encodings × number of slices ☐

60. The number of shots is calculated by:

a. TR × #PEs ☐
b. #PEs/ETL ☐
c. ETL/#PEs ☐
d. #PEs × NSA ☐

61. A single-shot FSE sequence is acquired when:

a. #PEs = 256 and ETL = 256 ☐
b. #PEs = 128 and ETL = 256 ☐
c. #PEs = 256 and ETL = 128 ☐
d. #PEs = 256 and ETL = 64 ☐

62. A multi-shot FSE sequence is acquired (with four shots) when:

a. #PEs = 256 and ETL = 256 ☐
b. #PEs = 128 and ETL = 256 ☐
c. #PEs = 256 and ETL = 128 ☐
d. #PEs = 256 and ETL = 64 ☐

63. To keep scan time at a minimum, diffusion imaging is typically performed with:

a. Single-shot EPI acquisition ☐
b. Single-shot FSE acquisition ☐
c. Multi-shot (two-shot) EPI acquisition ☐
d. Multi-shot (four-shot) EPI acquisition ☐

Data manipulation

64. The technique whereby a portion of the lines of k-space are "sampled" and "filled" and the remaining lines are interpolated is known as all of the following EXCEPT:

a. Half Fourier ☐
b. Partial Fourier ☐
c. Fractional Fourier ☐
d. Interleaved acquisition ☐

65. In a 3D acquisition, the slices are produced by:

a. A phase-encoding gradient applied in the slice selection direction ☐
b. Multiple 180° pulses along the slice selection direction ☐
c. Sampling multiple lines of K space per pulse sequence repetition ☐
d. Very accurate RF pulses ☐

66. The scan time for a 3D (or volume) acquisition is given by:

a. $TR \times NSA \times$ bandwidth $\times$ slice thickness ☐
b. $TR \times NSA \times$ number of phase encodings $\times$ number of slabs ☐
c. $TR \times NSA \times$ number of phase encodings $\times$ echo train length ☐
d. $TR \times NSA \times$ number of phase encodings $\times$ number of slices ☐

67. One direction in k-space represents phase, while the other represents:

a. Position ☐
b. Intensity ☐
c. Contrast ☐
d. Frequency ☐

68. With conventional spin echo each "line" of k-space is filled in each:

> **a.** Frequency-encoding period ☐
> **b.** TE period ☐
> **c.** TR period ☐
> **d.** Excitation period ☐

69. The top portion of k-space is a mirror image of the:

> **a.** Right ☐
> **b.** Left ☐
> **c.** Top ☐
> **d.** Bottom ☐

70. Acquiring half of the phase views of k-space and then interpolating the data for the other half is a technique known as:

> **a.** Zero fill ☐
> **b.** Fast spin echo ☐
> **c.** Half Fourier ☐
> **d.** Power scanning ☐

71. With a fast spin echo sequence utilizing an eight echo train length (ETL), the number of lines of k-space filled during each TR will be:

> **a.** 4 ☐
> **b.** 2 ☐
> **c.** 12 ☐
> **d.** 8 ☐

72. To create a projection image in MRA, the technique most commonly employed is:

> **a.** Multiplanar reconstruction ☐
> **b.** Region of interest calculation ☐
> **c.** Maximum intensity pixel ☐
> **d.** Summation pixel projection ☐

73. To evaluate the circle of Willis (COW), 3D TOF MRA sequences are acquired and displayed as an axial view of all of the vasculature. This image is known as:

> **a.** Multiplanar reconstruction ☐
> **b.** Segmented image ☐
> **c.** Minimum intensity pixel ☐
> **d.** Collapsed Image ☐

74. To evaluate the circle of Willis (COW), 3D TOF MRA sequences are acquired and background tissue is "carved out" to provide better visualization of the intracranial vasculature. This step is known as:

    a. Multiplanar reconstruction ☐
    b. Segmenting ☐
    c. Maximum intensity pixel ☐
    d. Collapsed Image ☐

75. Creating additional images in various planes from a 3D dataset is accomplished by a technique known as:

    a. Multiplanar reformatting ☐
    b. Region of interest calculation ☐
    c. Maximum intensity pixel ☐
    d. Summation pixel projection ☐

76. In order to produce a high-quality reformatted image, the:

    a. Acquisition voxel should be as rectangular as possible ☐
    b. Patient must hold their breath for the entire scan ☐
    c. Acquisition voxel should be isotropic ☐
    d. Acquisition voxel should be anisotropic ☐

77. Collecting the low frequency (high amplitude signal) data points in k-space at the start of the scan (in a rectilinear fashion) is known as:

    a. Linear ☐
    b. Centric ☐
    c. Elliptic centric ☐
    d. Reverse centric ☐

78. Collecting the low frequency (high amplitude signal) data points in k-space at the start of the scan (in a spiral fashion) is known as:

    a. Linear ☐
    b. Centric ☐
    c. Elliptic centric ☐
    d. Reverse centric ☐

79. During dynamic enhanced imaging for vasculature or visceral structures, contrast is administered and k-space is filled with _____ to ensure that the contrast enhancement is well visualized.

- **a.** Linear ☐
- **b.** Centric ☐
- **c.** Reverse centric ☐
- **d.** Reverse linear ☐

80. The high-frequency (low amplitude) data points in k-space provide:

- **a.** The bulk of the image's contrast ☐
- **b.** The majority of the image's signal ☐
- **c.** For a reduced noise contribution ☐
- **d.** Edge detail (spatial resolution) ☐

81. During contrast-enhanced imaging of the abdominal organs, images are acquired without and with gadolinium (Gd) enhancement. To better visualize contrast enhancement, _____ can be performed.

- **a.** Multiplanar reconstruction ☐
- **b.** Subtraction ☐
- **c.** Region of interest calculation ☐
- **d.** Maximum intensity pixel ☐

82. A 3D dataset can be reconstructed to display "what appears to be" a 3D image of the anatomy. This technique is known as:

- **a.** Multiplanar reconstruction (MPR) ☐
- **b.** Region of interest calculation (ROI) ☐
- **c.** Subtraction ☐
- **d.** Volume rendering (VR) ☐

83. The evaluation of cardiac function can be provided by any or all of the following EXCEPT:

- **a.** Cardiac ciné ☐
- **b.** Multiphase imaging ☐
- **c.** Perfusion imaging ☐
- **d.** Short axis single slice, single phase ☐

84. The technique by which signal data is transformed from a plot of signal intensity over time to a plot of signal intensity over frequency is known as:

    a. Fourier transformation ☐
    b. Chemical shift ☐
    c. Parts per million ☐
    d. Volume rendering ☐

85. The technique by which signal data is modified from the "time domain" to the "frequency domain" is known as:

    a. Fourier transformation ☐
    b. Chemical shift ☐
    c. Parts per million ☐
    d. Volume rendering ☐

86. Fourier transformation converts signal data from the FID into the spectrum.

    a. True ☐
    b. False ☐

87. Fourier transformation is performed in the:

    a. Fourier transformer ☐
    b. Array processor ☐
    c. K-spacer ☐
    d. RF amplifier ☐

88. Cardiac analysis performed with a technique using SAT bands to assess wall motion is known as:

    a. Myocardial tagging ☐
    b. Four-chamber imaging ☐
    c. Short-axis imaging ☐
    d. Cardiac gating ☐

Special procedures

89. Normal blood flow (demonstrated by a parabolic blood flow profile) is known as:

    a. Laminar flow ☐
    b. Accelerated flow ☐
    c. Vortex flow ☐
    d. Turbulent flow ☐

90. Blood flow at the area of a stenosis (vascular narrowing) is known as:

- **a.** Laminar flow ☐
- **b.** Accelerated flow ☐
- **c.** Vortex flow ☐
- **d.** Turbulent flow ☐

91. The swirling blood flow that occurs just past the area of a stenosis is known as:

- **a.** Laminar flow ☐
- **b.** Accelerated flow ☐
- **c.** Vortex flow ☐
- **d.** Turbulent flow ☐

92. Normal blood flow is known as:

- **a.** Laminar flow ☐
- **b.** Accelerated flow ☐
- **c.** Vortex flow ☐
- **d.** Turbulent flow ☐

93. A major advantage of MRA over conventional angiography is that:

- **a.** Images with both heavy T1 and T2 weighting can be produced ☐
- **b.** Multiple views can be produced from a single acquisition ☐
- **c.** Much smaller catheters are used ☐
- **d.** Less ionizing radiation is used ☐

94. The MRA sequence that is least sensitive to slow flow is:

- **a.** 3D phase contrast MRA (PC MRA) ☐
- **b.** 3D time of flight (TOF) ☐
- **c.** 2D PC ☐
- **d.** 2D TOF ☐

95. The MRA sequence that is most sensitive to smaller vessels is:

- **a.** 3D phase contrast MRA (PC MRA) ☐
- **b.** 3D time of flight (TOF) ☐
- **c.** 2D PC ☐
- **d.** 2D TOF ☐

96. The MRA sequence that is sensitive to flow direction is:

    a. 3D phase contrast MRA (PC MRA) ☐
    b. 3D time of flight (TOF) ☐
    c. 2D TOF ☐
    d. Multislice vascular ☐

97. The MRA sequence that can be made sensitive to any flow velocity is:

    a. 3D phase contrast MRA (PC MRA) ☐
    b. 3D time of flight (TOF) ☐
    c. 2D TOF ☐
    d. Multislice vascular ☐

98. The signal intensity on TOF MRA sequences is related to:

    a. Gadolinium ☐
    b. Flow-related enhancement ☐
    c. Velocity-induced phase shift ☐
    d. Restricted diffusion ☐

99. The signal intensity on PC MRA sequences is related to:

    a. Gadolinium ☐
    b. Flow-related enhancement ☐
    c. Velocity-induced phase shift ☐
    d. Restricted diffusion ☐

100. The signal intensity on diffusion sequences is related to:

    a. Gadolinium ☐
    b. Flow-related enhancement ☐
    c. Velocity-induced phase shift ☐
    d. Amount of diffusion ☐

101. The removal of signal from vessels in an MRA sequence is achieved by:

    a. Gradient moment nulling ☐
    b. Spatial presaturation ☐
    c. Spectral presaturation ☐
    d. a and b ☐

102. The following is (are) important in MRA sequences to minimize the loss of signal due to dephasing within a voxel:

> **a.** Long TR ☐
> **b.** Small voxels ☐
> **c.** Short TE ☐
> **d.** b and c ☐

103. Blood flow velocities are greatest:

> **a.** Further away from the heart ☐
> **b.** At a vessel wall ☐
> **c.** At the center of a vessel ☐
> **d.** In a 3D time of flight sequence ☐

104. Single-order gradient moment nulling does not compensate for:

> **a.** Accelerated flow ☐
> **b.** Reverse flow ☐
> **c.** Constant velocity flow ☐
> **d.** a and b ☐

105. In a spin echo sequence, flowing blood is normally seen as a signal void because the:

> **a.** TE is too long to image flow ☐
> **b.** Repetition times used in spin echo sequences are too long to image flow ☐
> **c.** 90° pulse and 180° pulse are both slice selective ☐
> **d.** Flip angle is always 90° ☐
> **e.** a and c ☐

106. In a vessel with a plaque producing a high degree of stenosis, the velocity of the blood flow in the center point of the stenosis is:

> **a.** Increased ☐
> **b.** Decreased ☐
> **c.** Reversed ☐
> **d.** Unaffected ☐

107. In a time of flight sequence, the tissue is HYPOintense relative to flowing blood because of the:

    a. T2 effects ☐
    b. T2* effects ☐
    c. Saturation effects ☐
    d. Inhomogeneities ☐

108. In a time of flight sequence, flowing blood is HYPERintense relative to stationary tissue because of the:

    a. T2 effects ☐
    b. Coil being used ☐
    c. Saturation pulse used ☐
    d. Flow-related enhancement ☐

109. Phase-contrast techniques produce images in which the signal intensity within the vessel is dependent on (among other parameters) the:

    a. Velocity of the flowing blood ☐
    b. T1 of the tissue ☐
    c. FOV selected ☐
    d. Number of phase-encoding views ☐

110. In a phase-contrast technique, it is possible to use the data to determine the:

    a. Exact size of the vessel lumen ☐
    b. Direction of blood flow ☐
    c. Temporal displacement of the vessel ☐
    d. Percentage stenosis of a lesion ☐

111. A major advantage of 3D time of flight techniques over 2D time of flight is the ability to:

    a. Determine blood flow velocities ☐
    b. Shorten imaging time ☐
    c. Visualize smaller vessels ☐
    d. Reduce the signal intensity from stationary tissue ☐

112. A major advantage of a 2D time of flight sequence over a 3D time of flight sequence is the ability to:

a. Image a larger area without saturation of the flowing blood ☐
b. Determine the percentage stenosis in the presence of a lesion ☐
c. Better image reverse flow ☐
d. Image a clot without showing the slower flow around it ☐

113. Cardiac ciné acquisitions typically utilize:

a. An inversion recovery pulse sequence ☐
b. A spin echo pulse sequence ☐
c. A gradient echo pulse sequence ☐
d. A fast spin echo pulse sequence ☐

114. Each "frame" of a cardiac ciné sequence displays the heart:

a. In various imaging planes ☐
b. With varying degrees of spatial resolution ☐
c. From a slightly different viewpoint ☐
d. In different phases of the cardiac cycle ☐

115. Ciné (kinematic) studies are often performed on various joints. The main purpose of such a study is to:

a. Visualize motion and function ☐
b. Visualize blood flow ☐
c. Measure muscle strength ☐
d. Impress referring physicians ☐

116. Which of the following would result in an image with the greatest amount of diffusion-weighting?

a. b-value 750 ☐
b. b-value 450 ☐
c. b-value 825 ☐
d. b-value 1100 ☐

117. The main purpose of producing/calculating an ADC map (image) is to:

a. Reduce the contribution from diffusion effects ☐
b. Eliminate the T2 shine-through ☐
c. Increase SNR ☐
d. Reduce T1 weighting ☐

118. Changing the b-value alters the:

> **a.** Amplitude, timing, and/or duration of the diffusion gradients ☐
> **b.** Amplitude of the phase-encoding gradient ☐
> **c.** Length of the readout gradient ☐
> **d.** Spatial resolution ☐

119. When performing a dynamic perfusion exam of the brain utilizing a gadolinium-based MR contrast agent, the result of the T2* shortening is:

> **a.** Increased MR signal ☐
> **b.** Reduced MR signal ☐
> **c.** Increased acquisition time ☐
> **d.** Increased chemical shift artifact ☐

120. The basic MR principle with regard to MR spectroscopy is:

> **a.** Faraday's law of induction ☐
> **b.** Chemical shift ☐
> **c.** Flow-related enhancement ☐
> **d.** The BOLD effect ☐

121. Having acquired a 3D TOF, when producing an MRA projection image set using the MIP technique, which of the following can appear bright and therefore the same as flow within a vessel?

> **a.** Tissues with long T2-relaxation times ☐
> **b.** Tissues or substances with extremely short T1-relaxation times ☐
> **c.** Polycystic astrocytoma ☐
> **d.** Any substance with an extremely short T2-relaxation time ☐

122. The intrinsic contrast mechanism with regard to fMRI is:

> **a.** Faraday's law of induction ☐
> **b.** Chemical shift ☐
> **c.** Flow-related enhancement ☐
> **d.** The BOLD effect ☐

123. All of the techniques below can be utilized to optimally time the start of a contrast-enhanced MRA EXCEPT:

a. Automated bolus detection ☐
b. Test bolus ☐
c. Centric k-space filling ☐
d. Real-time/fluoro triggering ☐

124. In order to reconstruct an image acquired using parallel imaging, which of the following may be required?

a. Test bolus ☐
b. Reference or calibration scan ☐
c. Back projection ☐
d. Half-Fourier acquisition ☐

125. When using parallel imaging to reduce acquisition times, which of the following is always true?

a. Scan time is reduced and spatial resolution is increased ☐
b. Spatial resolution is reduced the greater the acceleration factor selected ☐
c. SNR is not affected unless the acceleration factor is greater than 2 ☐
d. SNR is reduced and spatial resolution is unaffected ☐

Sequence parameters and options

126. The time between excitation pulses is known as the:

a. TI ☐
b. TE ☐
c. TR ☐
d. PR ☐

127. In a spin echo sequence, the time between the 90° pulse and the 180° pulse is:

a. TE ☐
b. TR ☐
c. TI ☐
d. ½ TE ☐

128. Presaturation pulses are often used to:

> **a.** Improve spatial resolution ☐
> **b.** Reduce flow artifacts ☐
> **c.** Reduce scan time ☐
> **d.** Turn flowing blood bright ☐

129. The presaturation pulses usually occur:

> **a.** Prior to the excitation pulse ☐
> **b.** After the 180° pulse ☐
> **c.** Between the 90° and 180° pulses ☐
> **d.** Prior to the TE ☐

130. Gradient echo sequences use flip angles:

> **a.** Less than 90° ☐
> **b.** That vary between pulse repetitions ☐
> **c.** To control saturation effects ☐
> **d.** To reduce SAR for larger patients ☐

131. Complete saturation is a condition where:

> **a.** Not enough time is given to allow the T2 decay to complete ☐
> **b.** The image becomes brighter ☐
> **c.** Longitudinal magnetization is not allowed to recover between excitations ☐
> **d.** Proton density effects predominate ☐

132. Increasing the TE:

> **a.** Increases the contrast based on T2-relaxation times of the tissues ☐
> **b.** Reduces the contrast based on T2-relaxation times of the tissues ☐
> **c.** Reduces the contrast based on T1-relaxation times of the tissues ☐
> **d.** a and c ☐

133. Reducing the TR down to or below the T1-relaxation time of the tissue:

> **a.** Decreases the signal-to-noise ratio (SNR) of the image ☐
> **b.** Reduces the contrast based on T2 relaxation times of the tissues ☐
> **c.** Increases saturation effects ☐
> **d.** a and c ☐

134. Reducing the TE:

> **a.** Increases the contrast based on T1 relaxation times ☐
> **b.** Increases the spin density contrast weighting ☐
> **c.** Reduces saturation effects ☐
> **d.** Reduces contrast based on T2 relaxation times ☐

135. As the TR increases:

> **a.** SNR increases up to a point ☐
> **b.** SNR decreases ☐
> **c.** SNR is not affected by TR ☐
> **d.** TE increases ☐

136. As the TE increases:

> **a.** SNR increases ☐
> **b.** SNR decreases ☐
> **c.** SNR is not affected by TE ☐
> **d.** TR increases ☐

137. In a gradient echo sequence, reducing the flip angle while holding the TR constant reduces:

> **a.** T2* contrast weighting ☐
> **b.** Spin density contrast weighting ☐
> **c.** Saturation ☐
> **d.** Scan time ☐

138. In a 2D conventional spin echo multislice pulse sequence, scan time is given by the equation:

  a. Time × number of phase encodings (# PEs) × TR (time to repetition) ☐

  b. TR (time to repetition) × FOV (field of view) × number of signals averaged (NSA) ☐

  c. TR (time to repetition) × number of slices (#Sl) × number of signals averaged (NSA) ☐

  d. TR (time to repetition) × number of signals averaged (NSA) × number of phase encodings (#PEs) ☐

139. In an inversion recovery pulse sequence, image contrast is controlled by:

  a. TR and TE only ☐

  b. TI only ☐

  c. TI and TE only ☐

  d. TR, TE, and TI ☐

140. In an inversion recovery pulse sequence, the time between the initializing 180° pulse and the 90° pulse is known as:

  a. TE ☐

  b. TR ☐

  c. TI ☐

  d. T1 ☐

141. Another name for TI is:

  a. Alpha ☐

  b. Theta ☐

  c. Sigma ☐

  d. Tau ☐

142. A short T1 inversion recovery (STIR) sequence can suppress the signal from:

  a. Fat ☐

  b. Water ☐

  c. A gadolinium-enhancing lesion ☐

  d. a and c ☐

143. Decreasing the receiver bandwidth (narrow BW):

> **a.** Decreases the SNR ☐
> **b.** Inverts the SNR ☐
> **c.** Increases the SNR ☐
> **d.** Has no effect on the SNR ☐

144. Decreasing the receiver bandwidth (narrow BW):

> **a.** Increases chemical shift artifact ☐
> **b.** Inverts chemical shift artifact ☐
> **c.** Reduces chemical shift artifact ☐
> **d.** Has no effect on chemical shift artifact ☐

145. Decreasing the receiver bandwidth (narrow BW):

> **a.** Increases readout time ☐
> **b.** Inverts the readout time ☐
> **c.** Reduces readout time ☐
> **d.** Has no effect on the readout time ☐

146. Decreasing the receiver bandwidth (narrow BW):

> **a.** Decreases susceptibility artifact ☐
> **b.** Inverts susceptibility artifact ☐
> **c.** Increases susceptibility artifact ☐
> **d.** Has no effect on the susceptibility artifact ☐

147. Decreasing the receiver bandwidth (narrow BW):

> **a.** Decreases the number of slices ☐
> **b.** Inverts the number of slices ☐
> **c.** Increases the number of slices ☐
> **d.** Has no effect on the number of slices ☐

148. Increasing the receiver bandwidth (wide BW):

> **a.** Decreases the available ETL ☐
> **b.** Inverts the available ETL ☐
> **c.** Increases the available ETL ☐
> **d.** Has no effect on the available ETL ☐

149. The time during which the frequency encoding gradient is on:

    a. Increases with a reduction in receiver bandwidth ☐

    b. Decreases with a reduction in receiver bandwidth ☐

    c. Is not affected by a reduction in receiver bandwidth ☐

    d. Cannot be changed by a reduction in receiver bandwidth ☐

150. In a conventional spin echo multi-echo sequence, it is possible to create multiple images, each with different amounts of:

    a. T1 weighting ☐

    b. Phase encoding ☐

    c. T2 weighting ☐

    d. Spatial resolution ☐

151. The SNR will increase in a 3D sequence with an increase in:

    a. FOV ☐

    b. Number of slices ☐

    c. TE ☐

    d. a and b ☐

152. Between slices 2D acquisitions generally require:

    a. Wait time ☐

    b. Gradient refocusing ☐

    c. Gaps ☐

    d. An inversion pulse ☐

153. Doubling the number of signals averaged (NSA) will:

    a. Decrease the SNR ☐

    b. Increase the SNR by the square root of 2 ☐

    c. Double the SNR ☐

    d. Not affect the SNR ☐

154. Increasing the number of phase encodings will produce an image with:

- **a.** Increased voxel volume ☐
- **b.** Decreased voxel volume ☐
- **c.** An unchanged voxel volume ☐
- **d.** Higher SNR ☐

155. Reducing NSA will reduce the scan time and:

- **a.** Decrease the SNR ☐
- **b.** Increase the SNR by a factor of 1.41 ☐
- **c.** Not affect the SNR ☐
- **d.** Double the SNR ☐

156. Doubling the NSA will increase the SNR by a factor of:

- **a.** 2 ☐
- **b.** 4 ☐
- **c.** 1.6 ☐
- **d.** 1.41 ☐

157. Reducing the FOV by a factor of 2 will reduce the voxel volume by a factor of:

- **a.** $\sqrt{2}$ ☐
- **b.** 2 ☐
- **c.** 8 ☐
- **d.** 4 ☐

158. If a STIR sequence using a TR of 3000, a TE of 20, and a TI of 140 produces an image with dark fat and bright water. The contrast in such an image is primarily based on:

- **a.** Flow ☐
- **b.** T1 ☐
- **c.** T2 ☐
- **d.** Dephasing ☐

159. In choosing the direction of phase encoding, the technologist usually considers the direction in which the:

- **a.** Most signal is needed ☐
- **b.** Scan time will not be affected ☐
- **c.** Motion artifacts traverse the least tissue or areas of interest ☐
- **d.** Resolution will not be distorted ☐

160. A chemical or spectral fat suppression sequence will suppress the signal from fat based on the:

   a. Precessional frequency of fat ☐
   b. Amount of fat in the target slice ☐
   c. T2 relaxation time of fat ☐
   d. a and c ☐

161. Increasing slice thickness from 5 to 10 mm (by a factor of 2, i.e. 2 × thicker), the SNR:

   a. Increases by a factor of 2 ☐
   b. Increases by a factor of 4 ☐
   c. Is not affected ☐
   d. Decreases by a factor of 2 ☐

162. Increasing the number of phase encodings (matrix) from 128 to 256 (by a factor of 2), the SNR:

   a. Increases ☐
   b. Inverts ☐
   c. Is not affected ☐
   d. Decreases ☐

163. Gradient moment nulling is most effective when correcting for motion-induced signal loss from:

   a. Pulsatile flow ☐
   b. No flow ☐
   c. Slow constant flow ☐
   d. Magnetic field inhomogeneities ☐

164. To rephase the signal from moving spins, gradient moment nulling techniques use a:

   a. RF pulse ☐
   b. Gradient ☐
   c. Series of short rapid pulses that are strategically timed ☐
   d. Flow encoding gradient ☐

165. Using a conventional spin echo multislice sequence, the number of slices allowed when increasing the TR:

  a. Decreases　☐
  b. Is not affected　☐
  c. Increases by a factor of TR/TE　☐
  d. Doubles　☐

166. Using a conventional spin echo multislice sequence, the number of slices allowed when increasing the TE from 20 to 40 ms:

  a. Decreases　☐
  b. Is not affected　☐
  c. Increases by a factor of TR × TE　☐
  d. Doubles　☐

167. Using a 3D acquisition, the number of slices allowed when increasing the TR:

  a. Decreases　☐
  b. Is not affected　☐
  c. Increases by a factor of TR/2　☐
  d. Doubles　☐

168. Using a 3D acquisition, increasing the number of slices from 64 to 128:

  a. Reduces the scan time　☐
  b. Has no effect on the scan time　☐
  c. Increases the scan time by a factor of 1.41　☐
  d. Doubles the scan time　☐

169. Increasing the matrix in the frequency direction from 256 to 512 will:

  a. Reduce the scan time　☐
  b. Have no effect on the scan time　☐
  c. Increase the scan time by a factor of 256/512　☐
  d. Double the scan time　☐

170. The effective TE in a fast spin echo pulse sequence determines the:

  a. Image contrast　☐
  b. Scan time　☐
  c. Spatial resolution　☐
  d. Number of frequency samples　☐

171. In a fast spin echo sequence, the central lines of k-space are associated with the:

    a. Image's spatial resolution   ☐
    b. TR   ☐
    c. Effective TE   ☐
    d. Scan time   ☐

172. When triggering a scan from the patient's ECG, the TR of the sequence is determined by the:

    a. Number of phase encodings selected   ☐
    b. Number of phases of the heart cycle being imaged   ☐
    c. Number of frequency encodings selected   ☐
    d. Patient's heart rate   ☐

173. Increasing TR:

    a. Increases scan time   ☐
    b. Inverts scan time   ☐
    c. Does not affect scan time   ☐
    d. Decreases scan time   ☐

174. Increasing TE:

    a. Increases scan time   ☐
    b. Inverts scan time   ☐
    c. Does not affect scan time   ☐
    d. Decreases scan time   ☐

175. Increasing the number of slices in a 2D acquisition:

    a. Increases scan time   ☐
    b. Inverts scan time   ☐
    c. Does not affect scan time   ☐
    d. Decreases scan time   ☐

176. For a given tissue with a given T1-relaxation time and TR, the flip angle, which will result in the maximum signal for that tissue, is:

    a. 90°   ☐
    b. 180°   ☐
    c. 45°   ☐
    d. the Ernst angle   ☐

177. Increasing the FOV:

- **a.** Increases scan time ☐
- **b.** Inverts scan time ☐
- **c.** Does not affect scan time ☐
- **d.** Decreases scan time ☐

178. Increasing the phase matrix:

- **a.** Increases scan time ☐
- **b.** Inverts scan time ☐
- **c.** Does not affect scan time ☐
- **d.** Decreases scan time ☐

179. Increasing the slice thickness:

- **a.** Increases scan time ☐
- **b.** Inverts scan time ☐
- **c.** Does not affect scan time ☐
- **d.** Decreases scan time ☐

180. Increasing the NSA:

- **a.** Increases scan time ☐
- **b.** Inverts scan time ☐
- **c.** Does not affect scan time ☐
- **d.** Decreases scan time ☐

181. Increasing the slice thickness:

- **a.** Increases SNR ☐
- **b.** Inverts SNR ☐
- **c.** Does not affect SNR ☐
- **d.** Decreases SNR ☐

182. Increasing the matrix:

- **a.** Increases SNR ☐
- **b.** Inverts SNR ☐
- **c.** Does not affect SNR ☐
- **d.** Decreases SNR ☐

183. Increasing the flip angle:

a. Increases SNR up to the Ernst angle ☐
b. Inverts SNR ☐
c. Does not affect SNR ☐
d. Always decreases SNR ☐

184. Reducing the ETL:

a. Increases scan time ☐
b. Inverts scan time ☐
c. Does not affect scan time ☐
d. Decreases scan time ☐

185. Reducing the TE:

a. Increases SNR ☐
b. Inverts SNR ☐
c. Does not affect SNR ☐
d. Decreases SNR ☐

186. Reducing the TE yields images with:

a. More T1 information ☐
b. Less T1 information ☐
c. More T2 information ☐
d. Less T2 information ☐

187. Increasing the TR yields images with:

a. More T1 information ☐
b. Less T1 information ☐
c. More T2 information ☐
d. Less T2 information ☐

188. Increasing the TE yields images with:

a. More T1 information ☐
b. Less T1 information ☐
c. More T2 information ☐
d. Less T2 information ☐

189. Reducing the TR yields images with:

> **a.** More T1 information ☐
> **b.** Less T1 information ☐
> **c.** More T2 information ☐
> **d.** Less T2 information ☐

190. Reducing the flip angle yields images with:

> **a.** More T1 information ☐
> **b.** Less T1 information ☐
> **c.** More T2 information ☐
> **d.** Less T2 information ☐

191. Increasing the flip angle yields images with:

> **a.** More T1 information ☐
> **b.** Less T1 information ☐
> **c.** More T2 information ☐
> **d.** Less T2 information ☐

Part C: Answers

1. **b**

2. **b**

3. **b**

    Figure C.3 shows examples of SE (top) and IR (below) sequences. Note that the IR sequence begins with a 180° RF pulse but the SE sequence begins with the 90° RF pulse.

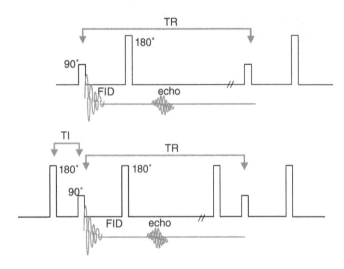

Figure C.3   Spin echo versus inversion recovery.

4. **d**

    FLAIR (fluid attenuated IR) sequences suppress the signal from fluid such as CSF within the ventricles of the brain. Anatomically, the anterior and posterior horns of the lateral ventricles are adjacent to the corpus callosum (white matter). When the patient has white matter disease (demyelinating disease) in the region of the corpus callosum, these lesions (plaques) appear bright on T2- and proton density-weighted images. When lesions are bright and fluid is bright, there is little or no distinction between structures. FLAIR sequences suppress the signal from fluid within the ventricles. In this case, the ventricle will be dark and the lesions bright. For this reason, FLAIR sequences are acquired for the evaluation of white matter disease that is near the ventricles (periventricular white matter disease).

5. **c**

    Figure C.4 demonstrates a simplified timing diagram for SE (left) and GrE (right) sequences. Note that the GrE sequence begins with a RF pulse with a flip angle that varies (depending upon the image contrast desired). Typically, GrE sequences use short TR to keep the scan time short. Regarding flip angle on GrE sequences,

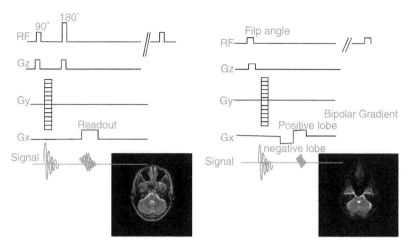

Figure C.4 Spin echo versus gradient echo.

a low flip angle (5–30°) is applied for T2* image contrast and a larger flip (up to 90°) for fast scans with T1 contrast. The SE sequence begins with the 90° RF pulse.

6. **d**

7. **d**

8. **c**

9. **d**

10. **c**

11. **a**
In a steady-state condition, there will be residual transverse magnetization at the time of the next excitation pulse.

12. **b**

13. **c**

14. **c**

15. **b**

16. **c**

17. **c**

18. **a**

19. **d**

20. **b**
Regarding questions 17–21: In a multi-echo spin echo pulse sequence, multiple echoes are used to produce multiple images with varying image contrast. In the

example shown in Figure C.1, 20 slice locations are acquired with a long TR and also with short TE (proton density) and long TE (T2 contrast) (question 17 and 18). Since T2 relaxation occurs at this time, images are acquired with more T2 information (produced by using a long TE) and less T2 information (produced by using a short TE) acquisitions (question 21). Although there are 20 slice locations prescribed, there will be 20 slices with short TE and 20 slices with long TE for a total of 40 images (question 17, 18, and 20). In this example there will be two slices acquired at the same location: one image with short TE and another with long TE values (question 19). In this case, one "set" of images is acquired (throughout the head) with a short TE (proton-density weighted) and another "set" of images is acquired (throughout the head) with a long TE (T2 weighted).

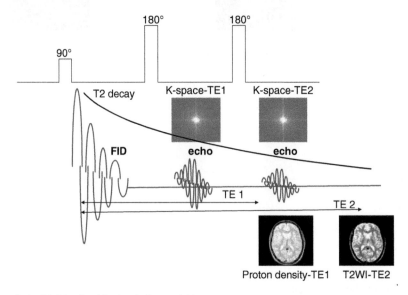

Figure C.1   Multi-echo (dual echo) acquisition.

During MR image acquisition, any combination of RF pulses produces an echo. An efficient combination of RF pulses includes the 90°/180° pulse combination. In multi-echo (ME) imaging and also in fast spin echo (FSE) imaging, each 180° RF pulse results in the creation of an echo. In ME imaging, each echo is used to produce an image with varying image contrast. In FSE imaging, each echo is used to fill one line in k-space. A FSE sequence acquired with the 'timing diagram' shown in Figure C.1 would produce a FSE sequence in half the time. In this example, k-space would be filled twice as fast as two lines are filled every TR period.

21. d

In a fast spin echo sequence, multiple echoes are used to fill multiple lines of k-space with each TR, thereby reducing scan time proportionally. In the example shown in Figure C.1, since two echoes are produced, two lines of k-space are filled with each TR, and scan time is reduced by a factor of 2. For example, a 12 minute spin echo sequence – acquired with FSE with an ETL of 2, yields a scan time of 6 minutes (question 23).

22. a

23. c

24. b

When discussing image acquisition and image formation, MR signal and MR gradients need to be understood. Many MR system users become confused by the term "amplitude", which merely means "strength". Therefore, it is possible to have a high amplitude gradient (strong gradient) and also a high amplitude signal (strong signal) and vice versa. Gradients can be applied with high amplitude (steep or strong gradient strength) or with low amplitude (flatter or weaker gradient strength).

MR signals are produced with high or low amplitude characteristics. A high amplitude signal is a strong or high signal; a low amplitude signal is a weak or low signal.

Low amplitude gradients (flatter gradients) produce low frequency/high amplitude echoes (strong signal). During spatial encoding, these high amplitude signals are encoded to the center lines of k-space. The lines in the center of k-space are weighted with image contrast and SNR information for the entire MR image. In FSE sequences, collecting these lines at the time of the effective TE will produce an image with the contrast and SNR of that particular TE.

High amplitude gradients (steeper gradients) produce high frequency/low amplitude echoes (weaker signals). These low amplitude signals are encoded to the "edges" of k-space. The lines to the edges of k-space are "weighted" with spatial resolution (or detail) information.

25. a

26. b

When FSE images are acquired with short effective TE values, the later (and lower amplitude or weaker) echoes are encoded for the edges of k-space. This combination of factors yields images with lower resolution due to blurring. To reduce blurring in FSE acquisitions (particularly with shorter TE values), images should be acquired with shorter ETL values (Hint: short TE/short ET).

However, when longer TE values are used, the earlier (and stronger) echoes are encoded to the edges of k-space, yielding less blurring and hence better image quality. For this reason, when FSE acquisitions are acquired with longer TE, then longer ET is acceptable for faster scan times (Hint: long TE/long ET).

27. b

This type of sequence may also be known as a spoiled gradient echo sequence. Gradient echo sequences were developed as "fast scan" or rapid imaging techniques. Typically, GrE sequences use short TR to keep scan time low. GrE sequences begin with a RF pulse with a flip angle that varies (depending upon the desired image contrast). Regarding flip angle on GrE sequences, flip angle "goes with" TR that goes with T1 relaxation. For this reason, a low flip angle (5–30°) is applied for "less T1 information", yielding T2* image. A larger flip (up to 90°) is applied for "more T1 information", yielding fast scans with T1 contrast.

28. c

When images are acquired with a spin echo (SE) acquisition, the 180° RF pulse is applied to create an echo and also to reduce the effects of characteristics such as susceptibility, inhomogeneity, and chemical shift (S-I-C, to name a few). When gradient echo (GrE) acquisitions are acquired, the echo is produced by the application of an additional gradient pulse. In this case, the effects of SIC have a significant impact on image quality. Furthermore, when multiple RF pulses are applied during GrE acquisitions, a condition known as steady state occurs. In a steady-state condition, residual transverse magnetization will exist at the time of the next excitation pulse. This steady-state effect produces T2* characteristics on GrE images. In this case, fast scans can only be produced with T2 (or T2*) image contrast (whereby fluid is bright). This technique is known as steady-state, T2* or coherent gradient echo imaging.

To reduce the steady-state (T2*) effect, a technique known as "spoiling" can be performed to allow for fast scans with T1 contrast. Spoiling can be performed by RF spoiling or gradient spoiling. RF spoiling occurs whereby additional RF pulses are randomized to "spoil" away the steady-state effect. This technique is known as spoiled gradient echo or incoherent gradient echo imaging. It is performed for rapid T1 imaging for dynamic enhanced imaging of the organs (liver, kidneys, etc.) and/ or dynamic enhanced MRA sequences.

29. b

30. a

31. a

32. d

33. a

Regarding questions 29–34: Gradient echo sequences are acquired with the use of a bipolar gradient. Since no 1800 RF pulse is applied on GrE sequences, susceptibility, inhomogeneity, and chemical shift (S-I-C) have a significant impact on image quality. Susceptibility artifact is also known as metal artifact. This artifact appears when metal is present (even in the form of iron in blood products). In this case, susceptibility artifacts allow for the determination of "blood" within or associated with lesions. Chemical shift occurs where fat and water "interface" in MR images. Chemical shift artifact is apparent on "out of phase" imaging. Inhomogeneity within the MR system or within the patient creates an overall degradation of image quality. Aliasing is not related to GrE imaging, but occurs when the anatomy is larger than the FOV. Aliasing is also known as fold-over or wrap around.

34. d

35. a

As the magnetic field strength increases (e.g. going from 0.5 T to 1.5 T), the "most challenging of both worlds happens". T1 relaxation time increases and T2 decay time decreases. Since TR goes with T1 and T1 changes with field strength, TR must be modified as field strength changes. Since TE goes with T2 and T2 changes (gets shorter) with field strength, TE must also be modified as field strength changes. Also, TI (the time to inversion or inversion time) goes with the T1 relaxation time, so as T1 increases the TI time should be increased to maintain image contrast.

36. b

37. c

38. d

39. b

40. a

41. c
Breaking down the acquisition of k-space into four shots results in four repetitions of the pulse sequence (four shots), each having an echo train of 64 echoes (256 phase/four shots). Given that all the other choices are single-shot techniques, the multi-shot option would result in the shortest train of echoes and thus the least susceptibility/distortion artifacts.

42. b

43. a

44. d

45. d

46. d
Parallel imaging is an imaging technique that is used to provide fast scans with unchanged spatial resolution at the cost of SNR. This technique is essentially associated with rectangular FOV imaging (to save scan time) without aliasing (which occurs when the FOV is smaller than the anatomy of interest). On parallel imaging, RF coils are used to "encode" MR signal. During parallel imaging, the RF coil spatially encodes the signal. For this reason, RF coils must be placed in a "parallel" configuration on the patient, e.g. in abdominal imaging, coils must be placed anterior and posterior on the abdomen (hence parallel to one another).

There are a number of parallel imaging techniques known as SENSE (SENSitivity Encoding), SMASH (SiMultaneous Acquisition of Spatial Harmonics) and GRAPPA (GeneRalized Autocalibrating Partially Parallel Acquisitions). Generally speaking, SENSE is said to be related to the image domain, SMASH to the frequency domain, and GRAPPA is a hybrid. There are also a number of vendor names for these techniques.

47. c
SENSE acquisitions are performed for rapid imaging with high resolution. SENSE sequences are performed whereby the RF coils are used to "encode" signal and hence maintain scan time. Sense imaging uses a low resolution "calibration" scan to provide information about RF signal detection.

48. c

49. c

50. c

51. d

52. a

53. a

54. a

55. d

56. c

57. b

58. d

59. d

60. b

61. a

62. d

63. a

64. d

When MR images are acquired, signal echoes are sampled and "encoded" to specific locations within k-space. For an imaging matrix of 256×256 there will be 256 lines and 256 points along each line (sampled and encoded into k-space). To save time during image acquisition, k-space filling can be "exploited". If a portion of k-space is filled (or half of k-space) is filled, scan time would be cut in half. This technique is known as half Fourier. Since half is a fraction, the technique is also known as fractional Fourier, and since a fraction is partially filled, it is also known as partial Fourier.

Interleaved acquisition is acquired to avoid cross-talk artifact. This technique provides a means to acquire every other slice (e.g. slice 1, 3, 5, and so on), and then comes back to fill the missing slices (e.g. slice 2, 4, 6, and so on).

65. a

66. d

67. d

The raw data from which an MR image is reconstructed is created by filling k-space. K-space consists of a series of lines determined by the phase-encoding gradient, with points along each line determined by the frequency encoding gradient.

68. c

69. d

The "top" portion of k-space is filled by the positive phase-encoding gradient applications. The "bottom" portion of k-space is filled after the application of the negative phase-encoding gradient steps. The positive phase-encoding gradients will shift the phase of the spins in the opposite direction to the shift produced by the negative phase-encoding steps, creating data that are a mirror image top to bottom as well as right to left.

70. c

71. d

72. c

73. d

74. b

75. a

Regarding Questions 73 – 76: TOF MRA techniques are acquired with the use of a 2D or 3D T1 gradient echo sequence. This sequence is acquired with TR and flip angle selections to suppress stationary tissues and allow for the visualization of flowing blood (within the vessels) after image acquisitions; reconstruction techniques are employed. The axial acquisitions are "stacked up" and then "collapsed". This technique allows for the visualization of all of the vessels that have been imaged. For example, if 3D, TOF MRA of the brain is acquired, the circle of Willis visualized.

This collapsed image can then be "carved out" to enable the visualization of the vessels. In this case, any stationary tissues with high signal (such as retro-orbital fat) can be "cut" out of the image. This technique is known as "segmenting".

Another option is to take the "stacked" axial images and send a "trace ray algorithm" through the volume of data, assigning the "maximum intensity" to the pixel of data that demonstrates "signal". This technique is known as MIP (maximum intensity pixel). Images then can be displayed in multiple imaging planes. This technique is known as multiplanar reconstruction (MPR).

76. c

The smallest unit of the 2D digital image is known as the pixel. The 3D volume element is known as the voxel. When images are acquired, with the intention of reconstruction into multiple imaging planes (MPR), image quality is improved with isotropic voxels. An isotropic voxel is essentially a "cube" whereby all sides are equal. When the voxel is isotropic, any and all reconstructed views will have the same spatial resolution.

Voxel size can be calculated from:

$$\text{FOV/matrix} = \text{slice thickness}$$

For example, if images are acquired with a 24-cm FOV and a 256×256 matrix, a slice thickness of 0.9375 will provide an isotropic voxel. The calculation is:

$$\text{FOV (24 cm} = 240 \text{ mm) divided by matrix (256)} = 0.9375 \text{ mm}$$

77. b

78. c

79. b

80. d
During spatial encoding, these high amplitude signals are encoded to the center lines of K space. The lines in the center of k-space are weighted with image contrast and SNR information for the entire MR image. In FSE sequences, collecting these lines at the time of the effective TE will produce an image with the contrast and SNR of that particular TE.

High amplitude gradients (steeper gradients) produce high frequency/low amplitude echoes (weaker signals). These low amplitude signals are encoded to the "edges" of k-space. The lines to the edges of k-space are "weighted" with spatial resolution (or detail) information.

81. b

82. d

83. d

84. a

85. a

86. a

87. b

88. a

89. a

90. b

91. c

92. d
Regarding questions 90–93: – Blood flow within the body does not have constant velocity, but (depending upon the vessel) can have a number of characteristics (Figure C.5). In a normal vessel, blood flow takes on a "parabolic" profile, whereby flow within the center of the vessel has higher velocity than flow toward the vessel walls. This is considered to be normal blood flow. The steepness of the parabola is determined by the blood flow velocity. High velocity flow will have a steep "bullet" shape or parabola (Figure C.5, lower left). Slow blood flow will have a flatter shape – known as "plug flow" (Figure C.5, upper left). The middle left image of Figure C.5 illustrates flow profiles for laminar (bottom), accelerated (at the area of stenosis – center of the vessel) and vortex flow (after the stenosis). On the TOF MRA (right), note the neck vessels and the area of stenosis in the internal carotid artery (arrow).

93. b

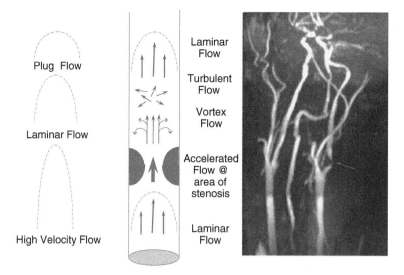

Figure C.5 Blood flow characteristics.

94. b

95. b

96. a

97. a

98. b

99. c

100. d

    Regarding questions 95–101: TOF MRA sequences use T1 gradient echoes with TR and flip angle selections to suppress the signal from stationary tissues, allowing for the visualization of flowing blood. The vascular signal on TOF MRA images is determined by flow-related enhancement (FRE). The vascular enhancement is related to the blood flow. 3D TOF is the best selection for the evaluation of smaller vessels and 2D TOF for the evaluation of slow flow.

    PC MRA sequences use T2 gradient echoes with parameter selections to suppress the signal from stationary tissues, allowing for the visualization of flowing blood. The vascular signal on PC MRA images is determined by velocity-induced phase shifts. PC MRA allows for the evaluation of flow velocity and flow direction. The VENC settings are chosen to evaluate slow flow (low VENC) or fast flow (high VENC) settings. PCMRA sequences use additional gradient pulses applied alongthe x, y, and z directions, with VENC (strength and duration of the gradients applied) settings.

    Diffusion imaging uses EPI sequences with additional gradient pulses applied along the x, y, and z directions (similar to PCMRA sequences). In this case a b-value is set. The b-value (similar to the VENC setting in PCMRA) determines the strength and duration of the gradient pulses. Tissues with restricted diffusion appear bright on diffusion imaging.

101. b

102. d

With longer TEs, more time is given for intravoxel dephasing, thereby reducing the signal from within the vessel. With larger voxels, inhomogeneities within the voxel are increased, and these also increase intravoxel dephasing and reduce signal intensity.

103. c

This is the case in what is known as laminar flow.

104. d

Single-order gradient moment nulling only compensates for first-order motion, such as flow with constant velocity.

105. e

Blood that is excited by the 90° pulse will have moved out of the slice by the time the 180° pulse has been applied. In order to produce a signal, tissue must receive both the 90° and the 180° pulses. Also, short TE allows less dephasing.

106. a

107. c

Time of flight effects will produce a low signal from the tissue yet a bright signal from the flowing blood (in a gradient echo sequence). The rapid repetition of the RF pulse, resulting from the selected TR time, will saturate the tissue, but fully magnetized (unsaturated) blood is continually being washed into the slice or imaging volume.

108. d

109. a

110. b

111. c

112. a

113. c

114. d

115. a

116. d

117. b

118. a

119. b

120. b

121. b

122. d

123. c

124. b

125. d

126. c

127. d

The TE is the time between the 90° pulse and the center of the echo. The 180° pulse occurs halfway between.

128. b

129. a

130. c

With gradient echo pulse sequences, increasing the flip angle will increase the saturation effects seen in the image and thus increase the T1 weighting.

131. c

132. a

133. d

134. d

135. a

136. b

137. c

138. d

139. d

140. c

141. d

142. d

A STIR sequence suppresses the signal from tissue, depending on that tissue's T1 relaxation time and the TI selected. Gadolinium shortens the T1 time of water molecules to close to the relaxation time of fat. With a short TI, the signal from both fat and gadolinium "enhancing" tissues can be suppressed.

143. c

144. a

145. a

146. c

147. a

148. d

149. a

150. c

151. d
Increasing the number of slices increases the slab thickness. This increases the amount of tissue excited, thus increasing the SNR. Increasing the FOV increases the voxel volume, which also increases the SNR.

152. c
Because the RF pulse profile is not perfect, when one slice is excited, the adjacent slices are slightly affected. This "cross-talk" causes a decrease in the SNR and contrast. Prescribing gaps between slices reduces cross-talk and thus improves image contrast and the SNR.

153. b
SNR is proportional to the square root of the total sampling time. Doubling the NSA would increase the SNR by a factor of 1.41 (square root of 2).

154. b

155. a

156. d

157. d
FOV affects the voxel volume in two dimensions – along the phase and frequency encoding axis of the image.

158. b

159. c

160. a

161. a

162. d

163. c

164. b

165. c

166. a

167. b

168. d

169. b

170. a

171. c

172. d

173. a

174. c

175. c

176. d

177. c

178. a

179. c

180. a

181. a

182. d

183. a

184. a

185. a

186. d

187. b

188. c

189. a

190. b

191. a

Physical Principles of Image Formation

MR Physics, Basic, Intermediate and Advanced Physics, Tissue Characteristics, Image Quality, and Types of MR Magnets, Coils, and Peripheral Equipment

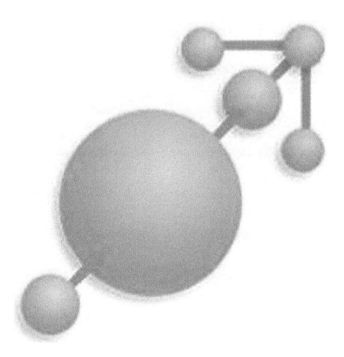

Introduction

The formation of an MR image is a complex process. The understanding of how images are formed requires a basic understanding of the system components (magnets, coils,

Review Questions for MRI, Second Edition. Carolyn Kaut Roth and William H. Faulkner.
© 2013 Carolyn Kaut Roth and William S. Faulkner. Published 2013 by Blackwell Publishing Ltd.

computers) and the physical principles of operation. Furthermore, MR technologists need to understand the fundamentals of the magnetic properties of tissues and how they behave in a magnetic field prior to, during, and following exposure to RF pulses. Finally, technologists must understand how artifacts are produced, learn to recognize them, and know how to correct for them. This understanding is crucial to their ability to consistently produce quality images for diagnosis.

Part D offers review questions and answers that pertain to the physical principles of image formation.

1. Instrumentation
   a. Electromagnetism
      - Faraday's law
      - Types of magnets (superconductive, permanent, resistive)
      - Magnetic field strength
   b. Radiofrequency system
      - Coil configuration
      - Transmit and receive coils
      - Transmit and receive bandwidth
      - Pulse profile
      - Phased array
   c. Gradient system
      - Coil configuration
      - Slew rate
      - Rise time
      - Duty cycle

2. Fundamentals
   a. Nuclear magnetism
      - Larmor equation
      - Precession
      - Gyromagnetic ratio
      - Resonance
      - RF pulse
      - Equilibrium magnetization
      - Energy state transitions
      - Phase coherence
      - Free induction decay (FID)
   b. Tissue characteristics
      - T1 relaxation
      - T2 relaxation
      - T2* (susceptibility)
      - Proton (spin) density
      - Flow
      - Diffusion
      - Perfusion

c. Spatial localization
- Vectors
- x, y, and z coordinate system
- Physical and logical gradient
- Slice select gradient
- Phase-encoding gradient
- Frequency (readout) gradient
- K-space (raw data)

3. Artifacts
   a. Cause and appearance of artifacts
   - Aliasing
   - Gibbs, truncation
   - Chemical shift
   - Magnetic susceptibility
   - Radiofrequency
   - Motion and flow
   - Partial volume averaging
   - Crosstalk

   b. Compensation for artifacts

4. Quality control
   a. Slice thickness
   b. Spatial resolution
   c. Contrast resolution
   d. Signal to noise
   e. Center frequency
   f. Transmit gain
   g. Geometric accuracy
   h. Equipment inspection (e.g. coils, cables, and door seals)

Questions 1–42 concern instrumentation, questions 43–106 fundamentals, questions 107–130 artifacts, and questions 131–147 quality control.

Part D: Questions

Instrumentation

1. Magnetic fields associated with MR imaging systems include the:
   1. Static magnetic field (B_0)
   2. RF (radiofrequency) field (B_1)
   3. Gradient field
   4. Gantry field

   a. 1 only ☐
   b. 1 and 2 only ☐
   c. 1, 2, and 3 only ☐
   d. 1, 2, 3, and 4 ☐

2. The MR system component that produces the B_0 field is the:

   a. Main magnet ☐
   b. Radiofrequency system ☐
   c. Gradient system ☐
   d. Shim system ☐

3. The MR system component that produces the B_1 field is the:

   a. Main magnet ☐
   b. Radiofrequency system ☐
   c. Gradient system ☐
   d. Shim system ☐

4. There are various types of magnets that can be used for MR imagers. These include:
   1. Permanent magnet
   2. Resistive magnet
   3. Hybrid magnet
   4. Superconducting magnet

   a. 1 only ☐
   b. 1 and 2 only ☐
   c. 1, 2, and 3 only ☐
   d. 1, 2, 3, and 4 ☐

5. The MR system component that provides a means for alignment (magnetization of proton spins) is the:

a. Main magnet ☐
b. Radiofrequency system ☐
c. Gradient system ☐
d. Shim system ☐

6. The MR system component that provides a means for excitation is the:

a. Main magnet ☐
b. Radiofrequency system ☐
c. Gradient system ☐
d. Shim system ☐

7. The MR system component that provides a means for spatial encoding is the:

a. Main magnet ☐
b. Radiofrequency system ☐
c. Gradient system ☐
d. Shim system ☐

8. The liquid cryogen(s) commonly used to maintain the magnet coil at superconducting temperature is(are):

a. Helium ☐
b. Hydrogen ☐
c. Nitrogen ☐
d. a and c ☐

9. Some systems use only one cryogen. In such systems, the cryogen is:

a. Nitrogen ☐
b. Hydrogen ☐
c. Helium ☐
d. Oxygen ☐

10. Faraday's law of induction states that if a loop of wire is moved through a magnetic field, _____ will be created in the wire.

- **a.** A magnetic wave ☐
- **b.** A voltage ☐
- **c.** Torque ☐
- **d.** Resonance ☐

11. The equation associated with Faraday's law of induction is:

- **a.** W/kg ☐
- **b.** b.
  $\omega 0 = B_0 \gamma$ ☐
- **c.** c.
  $\Delta B/\Delta T = \Delta V$ ☐
- **d.** Ppm ☐

12. According to Faraday's law of induction, the amount of current produced in a loop of wire moving through a magnetic field is proportional to the:

- **a.** Length of the wire ☐
- **b.** Strength of the magnetic field ☐
- **c.** Spin density of the wire ☐
- **d.** Time it takes for the magnetic field to reach full potential ☐

13. In a typical superconducting (cylindrical bore) magnet, the direction of the magnetic field is:

- **a.** Vertical ☐
- **b.** Horizontal ☐
- **c.** Around the flux lines ☐
- **d.** Hard to measure ☐

14. The direction of the magnetic field in a typical permanent magnet is:

- **a.** Vertical ☐
- **b.** Horizontal ☐
- **c.** Around the flux lines ☐
- **d.** Hard to measure ☐

15. To maintain the magnetic field of a resistive magnet, which of the following should be applied to the magnet coils?

> **a.** Water ☐
> **b.** Heat ☐
> **c.** Current ☐
> **d.** Cooling ☐

16. Magnetic field strength is measured in units of Tesla (T) and Gauss (G) whereby 1 T equals:

> **a.** 1 G ☐
> **b.** 1000 G ☐
> **c.** 10 000 G ☐
> **d.** 100 000 G ☐

17. 1.5 T equals:

> **a.** 10 000 G ☐
> **b.** 15 000 G ☐
> **c.** 30 000 G ☐
> **d.** 3000 G ☐

18. In a superconducting magnet, the magnetic field strength is increased by increasing the:

> **a.** Amount of cryogens ☐
> **b.** Temperature ☐
> **c.** Internal pressure ☐
> **d.** Turns of wire ☐

19. In a solenoid superconducting magnet, the direction of current flow affects the:

> **a.** Strength of the magnetic field ☐
> **b.** Direction of the magnetic field ☐
> **c.** Intensity of the magnetic field ☐
> **d.** Homogeneity of the magnetic field ☐

20. Permanent magnets with a vertical magnetic field use surface coils that are:

> **a.** Solenoids ☐
> **b.** Linear ☐
> **c.** Quadrature ☐
> **d.** Flat ☐

21. The transmit bandwidth of the RF pulse affects:

> **a.** Spatial resolution ☐
> **b.** Slice thickness ☐
> **c.** Image contrast ☐
> **d.** a and b ☐

22. In order to create a thin slice thickness, a _____ is used.
   1. Steep slice selection gradient
   2. High amplitude slice selection gradient
   3. Narrow transmit bandwidth (tBW)
   4. Narrow receiver bandwidth (rBW)

> **a.** 1 only ☐
> **b.** 1 and 2 only ☐
> **c.** 1, 2, and 3 ☐
> **d.** 1, 2, 3, and 4 only ☐

23. The receiver bandwidth affects:

> **a.** Chemical shift artifact ☐
> **b.** Slice thickness resolution ☐
> **c.** Signal-to-noise ratio (SNR) ☐
> **d.** a and c ☐

24. If a coil is improperly tuned, it will result in:

> **a.** A decrease in SNR ☐
> **b.** A reduction in voxel size ☐
> **c.** Patient burns ☐
> **d.** Resonance artifacts ☐

25. The gradient magnetic fields are:

> **a.** Always on ☐
> **b.** Superimposed over the main magnetic field ☐
> **c.** Used for contrast control ☐
> **d.** Controlled by RF pulses ☐

26. The timing of RF pulses during an MR pulse sequence:

> **a.** Controls image contrast ☐
> **b.** Spatially encodes the data ☐
> **c.** Shims the static magnetic field ☐
> **d.** a and b ☐

27. The B1 magnetic field is produced by a:

> **a.** Gradient coil ☐
> **b.** Shim coil ☐
> **c.** Radiofrequency coil ☐
> **d.** Magnet coil ☐

28. In an MRI system that uses shim coils, B_0 homogeneity is adjusted by:

> **a.** Changing current in the shim coil ☐
> **b.** Adding metal to different coils within the shim coil ☐
> **c.** Adding current to the gradient coils ☐
> **d.** Turning the shim coil off and on very rapidly ☐

29. Shimming in MRI is performed by all of the following EXCEPT:

> **a.** Changing current in the shim coil ☐
> **b.** Adding metal to different coils within the shim coil ☐
> **c.** Adding current to the gradient coils ☐
> **d.** Turning the shim coil off and on very rapidly ☐

30. Gradient strength (amplitude) is measured in units of:
> **1.** mT/M
> **2.** G/cm
> **3.** T/m/s
> **4.** μs
> **5.** %

> **a.** 1 only ☐
> **b.** 1 and 2 only ☐
> **c.** 3 only ☐
> **d.** 4 only ☐
> **e.** 5 only ☐

31. Gradient speed (rise time) is measured in units of:
  1. mT/M
  2. G/cm
  3. T/m/s
  4. μs
  5. %

  a. 1 only   ☐
  b. 1 and 2 only   ☐
  c. 3 only   ☐
  d. 4 only   ☐
  e. 5 only   ☐

32. Gradient speed (rise time) and strength (amplitude) is measured in units of:
  1. mT/M
  2. G/cm
  3. T/m/s
  4. μs
  5. %

  a. 1 only   ☐
  b. 1 and 2 only   ☐
  c. 3 only   ☐
  d. 4 only   ☐
  e. 5 only   ☐

33. The amount of time that a gradient is "permitted" to work is known as the duty cycle and is measured in units of:
  1. mT/M
  2. G/cm
  3. t/m/s
  4. μs
  5. %

  a. 1 only   ☐
  b. 1 and 2 only   ☐
  c. 3 only   ☐
  d. 4 only   ☐
  e. 5 only   ☐

34. The gradient strength is measured in units of:

> **a.** Amplitude ☐
> **b.** Slew rate ☐
> **c.** Duty cycle ☐
> **d.** Rise time ☐

35. The gradient characteristic that reflects both strength and speed is known as the:

> **a.** Amplitude ☐
> **b.** Slew rate ☐
> **c.** Duty cycle ☐
> **d.** Rise time ☐

36. Gradients can work for a period of time known as the:

> **a.** Amplitude ☐
> **b.** Slew rate ☐
> **c.** Duty cycle ☐
> **d.** Rise time ☐

37. Gradient characteristic for speed is known as the:

> **a.** Amplitude ☐
> **b.** Slew rate ☐
> **c.** Duty cycle ☐
> **d.** Rise time ☐

38. RF coil configurations include:
  1. Linear
  2. Quadrature
  3. Phase array
  4. Helmholtz
  5. Multichannel

> **a.** 1 only ☐
> **b.** 1 and 2 only ☐
> **c.** 1, 2, and 3 only ☐
> **d.** 1, 2, 3, and 4 only ☐
> **e.** 1, 2, 3, 4, and 5 ☐

39. RF coil configurations that use multiple coils with one single receiver include:
   1. Linear
   2. Quadrature
   3. Phase array
   4. Helmholtz
   5. Multichannel

   a. 1 only ☐
   b. 1 and 2 only ☐
   c. 3 and 5 only ☐
   d. 4 only ☐

40. RF coil configurations that use multiple coils with multiple receivers include:
   1. Linear
   2. Quadrature
   3. Phase array
   4. Helmholtz
   5. Multichannel

   a. 1 only ☐
   b. 1 and 2 only ☐
   c. 3 and 5 only ☐
   d. 4 only ☐

41. The sensitivity profile for a given coil is known as the:

   a. Pulse profile ☐
   b. Spectrum ☐
   c. FID ☐
   d. Echo ☐

42. RF coil configurations that use coils whereby the coil is configured with wires (or electronic components) that are perpendicular to one another are known as:
   1. Linear
   2. Quadrature
   3. Phase array
   4. Helmholtz
   5. Multichannel

   a. 1 and 2 only ☐
   b. 2 only ☐
   c. 3 and 5 only ☐
   d. 4 only ☐

Fundamentals

43. In the equation associated with Larmor Equation, B_0 stands for:

- **a.** Static magnetic field ☐
- **b.** Frequency ☐
- **c.** Gyromagnectic ratio ☐
- **d.** Voltage ☐

44. In the equation associated with Larmor Equation, ω_0 stands for:

- **a.** Static magnetic field ☐
- **b.** Frequency ☐
- **c.** Gyromagnectic ratio ☐
- **d.** Voltage ☐

45. In the equation associated with Larmor Equation, γ stands for:

- **a.** Static magnetic field ☐
- **b.** Frequency ☐
- **c.** Gyromagnectic ratio ☐
- **d.** Voltage ☐

46. A magnetic field strength of 0.5 T is equivalent to:

- **a.** 15 000 G ☐
- **b.** 5000 G ☐
- **c.** 1 G ☐
- **d.** 10 000 G ☐

47. A condition whereby there are MORE spins "in line" with the magnetic field than "opposed" is known as:

- **a.** Low energy ☐
- **b.** High energy ☐
- **c.** Thermal equilibrium ☐
- **d.** Excitation ☐

48. During thermal equilibrium there are:

- **a.** More spins in the low energy state ☐
- **b.** More spins in the high energy state ☐
- **c.** Equal number of spins in the low and high energy state ☐
- **d.** Less spins in the low energy state ☐

49. Proton spins that are "in line" with the static magnetic field (B_0) are referred to as all of the following EXCEPT:

> **a.** Spin up ☐
> **b.** Parallel ☐
> **c.** Low energy spins ☐
> **d.** High energy spins ☐

50. The microscopic magnetic field associated with the proton within the magnetic field is known as the:

> **a.** Free induction decay (FID) ☐
> **b.** Magnetic moment (μ) ☐
> **c.** Signal echo (SE) ☐
> **d.** Field of view (FOV) ☐

51. During thermal equilibrium, the vector that represents the "spin excess" is known as the:

> **a.** Free induction decay (FID) ☐
> **b.** Net magnetization vector (NMV) ☐
> **c.** Signal echo (SE) ☐
> **d.** Field of view (FOV) ☐

52. The RF pulse is applied to achieve a condition known as:

> **a.** Thermal equilibrium ☐
> **b.** Excitation ☐
> **c.** Relaxation ☐
> **d.** Scan timing ☐

53. During excitation, all of the following occur EXCEPT:

> **a.** Low energy spins enter the high energy state ☐
> **b.** Spins begin to precess "in phase" ☐
> **c.** The net magnetization is transferred into the transverse (x/y) plane ☐
> **d.** High energy spins return to the low energy state ☐

54. During relaxation, all of the following occur EXCEPT:

> **a.** Low energy spins enter the high energy state ☐
> **b.** High energy spins return to the low energy state ☐
> **c.** Spins begin to precess "out of phase" or lose phase coherence ☐
> **d.** The net magnetization recovers longitudinally ☐

55. T1 relaxation is also known as all of the following EXCEPT:

a. T1 recovery ☐
b. Spin lattice ☐
c. Longitudinal recovery or relaxation ☐
d. Spin–spin ☐

56. T2 relaxation is also known as:

a. T1 recovery ☐
b. Spin lattice ☐
c. Longitudinal recovery or relaxation ☐
d. Spin–spin ☐

57. T2 relaxation is also known as all of the following EXCEPT:

a. T2 decay ☐
b. Spin lattice ☐
c. Spin–spin ☐
d. Transverse relaxation ☐

58. T1 relaxation time is defined as when:

a. 76% of the longitudinal magnetization has regrown ☐
b. 63% of the longitudinal magnetization has regrown ☐
c. 63% of the transverse magnetization has regrown ☐
d. 76% of the tissue's magnetization has regrown ☐

59. T2 relaxation time is defined as when:

a. 76% of the longitudinal magnetization has decayed ☐
b. 63% of the longitudinal magnetization has decayed ☐
c. 63% of the transverse magnetization has decayed ☐
d. 76% of the tissue's magnetization has decayed ☐

60. Images acquired with a spin echo pulse sequence having a SHORT TR and TE values yield images known as (Figure D.1):

a. T1WI ☐
b. T2WI ☐
c. PDWI ☐
d. Diffusion images ☐

61. Images acquired with a spin echo pulse sequence having LONG TR and TE values yield images known as (Figure D.1):

    a. T1WI ☐
    b. T2WI ☐
    c. PDWI ☐
    d. Diffusion images ☐

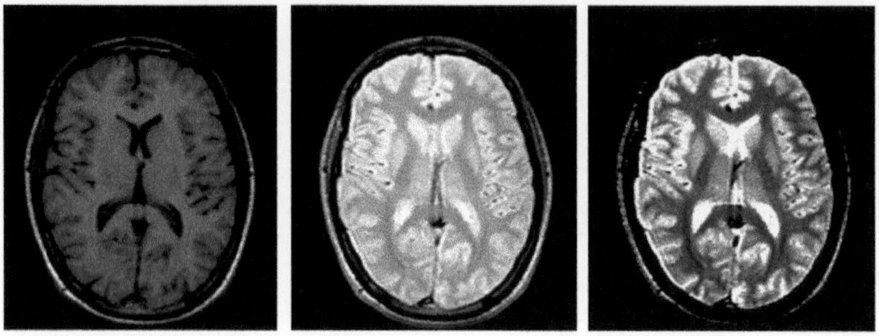

T1WI	PDWI	T2WI
Short TR	Long TR	Long TR
Short TE	Short TE	Long TE
Bright fat, short T1 time	Bright fat & water	Bright water, long T2 time

Figure D.1

62. Images acquired with a spin echo pulse sequence having LONG TR and SHORT TE values yield images known as (Figure D.1):

    a. T1WI ☐
    b. T2WI ☐
    c. PDWI ☐
    d. Diffusion images ☐

63. Spin density is another term for (Figure D.1):

    a. Nuclear density ☐
    b. Spin density ☐
    c. Proton density ☐
    d. b and c ☐

64. Spin density is determined by the (Figure D.1):

    a. Amount of excess spins in the low energy state at equilibrium ☐
    b. Amount of transverse magnetization at the time the echo is sampled ☐
    c. T1/T2 ☐
    d. Amount of excess spins in the high energy state at equilibrium ☐

65. Gradient echo (steady-state) sequences acquired with short TR and flip angle combinations along with a moderately long TE yield images with (Figure D.1):

  a. T1 contrast ☐
  b. T2 contrast ☐
  c. PD contrast ☐
  d. T2* contrast ☐

66. T2 + T2′ equals (Figure D.1):

  a. T1 ☐
  b. T2 ☐
  c. PD ☐
  d. T2* ☐

67. The LOGICAL gradient that is used for slice selection for the acquisition of an axial slice is the:

  a. x ☐
  b. y ☐
  c. z ☐
  d. A combination of gradients ☐

68. The PHYSICAL gradient that is used for slice selection for the acquisition of an axial slice is the:

  a. x ☐
  b. y ☐
  c. z ☐
  d. A combination of gradients ☐

69. The LOGICAL gradient that is used for slice selection for the acquisition of a sagittal slice is the:

  a. x ☐
  b. y ☐
  c. z ☐
  d. A combination of gradients ☐

70. The PHYSICAL gradient that is used for slice selection for the acquisition of an sagittal slice is the:

a. x ☐
b. y ☐
c. z ☐
d. A combination of gradients ☐

71. The LOGICAL gradient that is used for phase encoding for the acquisition of an axial slice of the abdomen is the:

a. x ☐
b. y ☐
c. z ☐
d. A combination of gradients ☐

72. The LOGICAL gradient that is used for phase encoding for the acquisition of an axial slice of the head is the:

a. x ☐
b. y ☐
c. z ☐
d. A combination of gradients ☐

73. The PHYSICAL gradient that is used for phase encoding for the acquisition of an axial slice of the abdomen is the:

a. x ☐
b. y ☐
c. z ☐
d. A combination of gradients ☐

74. The PHYSICAL gradient that is used for phase encoding for the acquisition of an axial slice of the head is the:

a. x ☐
b. y ☐
c. z ☐
d. A combination of gradients ☐

75. The receiver bandwidth is related to the slope of the:

- **a.** Frequency-encoding gradient ☐
- **b.** Phase-encoding gradient ☐
- **c.** Slice-selecting gradient ☐
- **d.** Transmitting gradient ☐

76. Following a 90° RF pulse, the signal that is created is called:

- **a.** Spin echo ☐
- **b.** Gradient echo ☐
- **c.** Free induction decay ☐
- **d.** FRE ☐

77. T2* is a result of dephasing due to a tissue's T2 time and:

- **a.** T1 ☐
- **b.** Susceptibility, inhomogeneities, and chemical shift ☐
- **c.** Molecular weight ☐
- **d.** a and b ☐

78. The peak signal strength of a spin echo is less than the initial signal strength of the free induction decay because of:

- **a.** T1 relaxation ☐
- **b.** T2* decay ☐
- **c.** Spin density changes ☐
- **d.** T2 relaxation ☐

79. An example of a dipole is:

- **a.** A hydrogen nucleus ☐
- **b.** A bar magnet ☐
- **c.** The earth ☐
- **d.** a, b, and c ☐

80. A vector has both direction and:

- **a.** Purpose ☐
- **b.** Current ☐
- **c.** Magnitude ☐
- **d.** A fractional equivalent force ☐

81. Hydrogen nuclei have a magnetic moment because they possess a property called:

> **a.** Inversion ☐
> **b.** Flux ☐
> **c.** Spin ☐
> **d.** Resonance ☐

82. When placed in a large static magnetic field, hydrogen nuclei:

> **a.** Align with the magnetic field ☐
> **b.** Align in either a parallel or antiparallel position ☐
> **c.** Oscillate ☐
> **d.** Relax ☐

83. Spins aligned in the antiparallel direction are in:

> **a.** An expanded energy state ☐
> **b.** A resonant condition ☐
> **c.** A high-energy state ☐
> **d.** A constant state of flux ☐

84. During thermal equilibrium, the spin excesses of individual hydrogen nuclei add to form:

> **a.** A rotating vector ☐
> **b.** An oscillating vector ☐
> **c.** A varying vector ☐
> **d.** A net magnetization vector ☐

85. The formula that describes the relationship between the static magnetic field and the precessional frequency of the hydrogen protons is the:

> **a.** Helmholtz relationship ☐
> **b.** Nyquist theorem ☐
> **c.** Larmor equation ☐
> **d.** Bloch equation ☐

86. To calculate the precessional frequency, the strength of the static magnetic field is multiplied by a constant known as the:

a. Gyromagnetic ratio ☐
b. Tau ☐
c. Alpha-1 ☐
d. Linear attenuation coefficient ☐

87. The condition reached within a few seconds of hydrogen being placed in a magnetic field is described as:

a. Resonance ☐
b. Free induction decay ☐
c. Phase coherence ☐
d. Thermal equilibrium ☐

88. During thermal equilibrium, the individual protons precess:

a. At the same frequency ☐
b. In phase ☐
c. Out of phase ☐
d. Slower ☐

89. In order for energy to transfer between systems, the two systems must be at the same:

a. Phase location ☐
b. Energy level ☐
c. Mass ☐
d. Resonant frequency ☐

90. Assuming a TR sufficient for full recovery of longitudinal magnetization, maximum signal is produced in the receiver coil when the net magnetization is tipped:

a. 180° ☐
b. 90° ☐
c. Away from the z axis ☐
d. Through the transverse plane ☐

91. In relation to the static magnetic field (B_0), the RF field (B_1) is oriented:

    a. Parallel ☐
    b. Perpendicular ☐
    c. At 180° ☐
    d. At 45° ☐

92. The RF energy used in MRI is classified as:

    a. Electromagnetic radiation ☐
    b. Ionizing radiation ☐
    c. Nonradiation energy ☐
    d. Investigational ☐

93. Immediately on the application of the 90° pulse, the precessing protons:

    a. All flip to the high energy state ☐
    b. Tip into the transverse plane ☐
    c. Begin to precess in phase ☐
    d. a and b ☐

94. The MR signal is produced by magnetization:

    a. Out of phase ☐
    b. In the longitudinal direction ☐
    c. Decayed ☐
    d. In the transverse plane ☐

95. Frequency can be defined by the:

    a. Rate of phase change per unit time ☐
    b. Phase/2 ☐
    c. Fourier equation ☐
    d. Amplitude of the signal ☐

96. Gradient magnetic fields are used to:

    a. Improve the SNR ☐
    b. Spatially encode the data ☐
    c. Transmit the RF pulse ☐
    d. Control the image contrast ☐

97. Slice thickness is controlled by:

a. Length of the gradient field ☐
b. Slope of the gradient ☐
c. Receiver bandwidth ☐
d. a and b ☐

98. The physical gradient along the bore of a superconducting magnet is the:

a. *x* gradient ☐
b. *x*, *y* gradient ☐
c. *y* gradient ☐
d. *z* gradient ☐

99. To produce a sagittal slice, the physical gradient used during the excitation pulse is the:

a. *z* gradient ☐
b. *y* gradient ☐
c. *x* gradient ☐
d. a and b ☐

100. The gyromagnetic ratio for hydrogen is:

a. 63.86 MHz/T ☐
b. 42.6 MHz/T ☐
c. 1 G/cm ☐
d. 4 W/kg ☐

101. In a 0.5-T imager, the precessional frequency of hydrogen is approximately:

a. 63.86 MHz ☐
b. 42.6 MHz ☐
c. 21.3 MHz ☐
d. 0.5 MHz ☐

102. The amount of RF energy necessary to produce a 45° flip angle is determined by the:

a. Coil being used ☐
b. Amplitude (power) and duration of the RF pulse ☐
c. Strength of the external magnetic field ☐
d. All of the above ☐

103. The gradient that varies in amplitude with each TR is the:

a. Phase-encoding gradient ☐
b. Frequency-encoding gradient ☐
c. Slice selecting gradient ☐
d. a and b ☐

104. The gradient that is on during the sampling of the echo is the:

a. Phase-encoding gradient ☐
b. Frequency-encoding gradient ☐
c. Slice-selecting gradient ☐
d. a and b ☐

105. K-space is:

a. The image in its natural state ☐
b. A negative of an MR image ☐
c. The raw data from which an MR image is created ☐
d. What comes after J space ☐

106. Multiple coil elements combined with multiple receiver channels is a:

a. Quadrature coil ☐
b. Surface coil ☐
c. Linear coil ☐
d. Phased array coil ☐

Artifacts

107. The superimposition of signal that occurs when a LARGE FOV is acquired is known as:

a. Wrap around ☐
b. Fold over ☐
c. Aliasing ☐
d. Partial volume averaging ☐

108. The superimposition of signal that occurs when a SMALL FOV is acquired is known as all of the following EXCEPT:

    a. Wrap around ☐
    b. Fold over ☐
    c. Aliasing ☐
    d. Partial volume averaging ☐

109. Motion is seen as a smearing in the:

    a. Frequency-encoding direction ☐
    b. Phase-encoding direction ☐
    c. Slice-selection direction ☐
    d. z axis direction ☐

110. Aliasing occurs because tissue outside the selected FOV is:

    a. Undersampled ☐
    b. Oversampled ☐
    c. Not sampled ☐
    d. Too large ☐

111. In order to compensate for aliasing:

    a. The scan can be shortened ☐
    b. The FOV can be enlarged ☐
    c. An oversampling technique can be employed ☐
    d. b and c ☐

112. Gibbs, or truncation, artifact is seen as:

    a. Tissue that looks very similar to aliased tissue ☐
    b. A bright pixel in the center of the image ☐
    c. Dark lines between fat and water interfaces within the image ☐
    d. High and low signal intensity bands ☐

113. To correct for Gibbs artifact the:

    a. Number of phase encodings is decreased ☐
    b. Number of phase encodings is increased ☐
    c. FOV is increased ☐
    d. TE is decreased ☐

114. Chemical shift occurs because the:

a. System is undersampling the fat and water molecules ☐
b. SNR is low ☐
c. Fat and water precess at different frequencies ☐
d. Tissue is undersampled in the frequency direction ☐

115. Chemical shift becomes more obvious as the:

a. Transmitter bandwidth is increased ☐
b. Receiver bandwidth is decreased ☐
c. Receiver bandwidth is increased ☐
d. Field strength of the magnet decreases ☐

116. Magnetic susceptibility effects are more prominent with:

a. Gradient echo sequences ☐
b. Spin echo sequences ☐
c. Fast spin echo sequences ☐
d. Inversion recovery sequences ☐

117. Magnetic susceptibility effects are less prominent with:

a. Gradient echo sequences ☐
b. Spin echo sequences ☐
c. Fast spin echo sequences ☐
d. Inversion recovery sequences ☐

118. Susceptibility effects can be reduced by:

a. Reducing the FOV ☐
b. Reducing the TR ☐
c. Reducing the TE ☐
d. a and c ☐

119. A leak in the RF shielding can appear as a:

a. Bright spot in the center of the image ☐
b. "Zipper" artifact in the frequency direction ☐
c. Wet spot on the image ☐
d. Ghost along the image's edge ☐

120. Flow artifacts can be reduced by:

a. Gradient moment nulling ☐
b. Spatial presaturation pulses ☐
c. Shortening the TE ☐
d. All of the above ☐

121. A decrease in voxel volume leads to a decrease in:

a. Chemical shift ☐
b. Aliasing ☐
c. Partial volume averaging ☐
d. a and c ☐

122. As FOV increases, partial volume averaging:

a. Increases ☐
b. Decreases ☐
c. Stays the same ☐
d. Is not affected ☐

123. As slice thickness increases, partial volume averaging:

a. Increases ☐
b. Decreases ☐
c. Stays the same ☐
d. Is not affected ☐

124. As matrix increases, partial volume averaging:

a. Increases ☐
b. Decreases ☐
c. Stays the same ☐
d. Is not affected ☐

125. As TR increases, partial volume averaging:

a. Increases ☐
b. Decreases ☐
c. Stays the same ☐
d. Is not affected ☐

126. Respiratory artifacts can be reduced by:

   a. Respiratory gating ☐
   b. Respiratory triggering ☐
   c. Increasing the number of signals averaged ☐
   d. All of the above ☐

127. Motion artifact occurs due to period and/or aperiodic motion, whereby respiratory motion is an example of:

   a. Periodic motion ☐
   b. Aperiodic motion ☐
   c. Random motion ☐
   d. Daily motion ☐

128. Motion artifact occurs due to period and/or aperiodic motion, whereby cardiac motion is an example of:

   a. Periodic motion ☐
   b. Aperiodic motion ☐
   c. Random motion ☐
   d. Daily motion ☐

129. Motion artifact occurs due to period and/or aperiodic motion, whereby patient movement is an example of:

   a. Periodic motion ☐
   b. Aperiodic motion ☐
   c. Pulsatile motion ☐
   d. Daily motion ☐

130. Motion artifact occurs due to period and/or aperiodic motion, whereby peristaltic motion is an example of:

   a. Periodic motion ☐
   b. Aperiodic motion ☐
   c. Pulsatile motion ☐
   d. Daily motion ☐

Quality control

131. If the slice thickness is reduced by a factor of 2, the factor by which the NSA must be increased to maintain the same SNR (all other factors remaining constant) is:

    a. 8 ☐
    b. 1.41 ☐
    c. 4 ☐
    d. 2 ☐

132. If the slice thickness is increased by a factor of 2 (from 5 to 10 mm thickness), the SNR (all other factors remaining constant):

    a. Increases by the square root of two ☐
    b. Increases by a factor of 2 ☐
    c. Reduces by a factor of 2 ☐
    d. Reduces by a factor of the square root of 2 ☐

133. If the slice thickness increases, the SNR (all other factors remaining constant):

    a. Increases ☐
    b. Decreases ☐
    c. Stays the same ☐
    d. Is not affected ☐

134. If the slice thickness increases, the spatial resolution (all other factors remaining constant):

    a. Increases ☐
    b. Decreases ☐
    c. Stays the same ☐
    d. Is not affected ☐

135. Changing the size of the voxel in the frequency direction will:

    a. Double the scan time ☐
    b. Decrease the scan time ☐
    c. Have no effect on the scan time ☐
    d. Increase the scan time by a factor of 0.5 ☐

136. Factors that affect contrast (contrast to noise or contrast resolution) include all of the following EXCEPT:

   a. TR ☐
   b. TE ☐
   c. TI ☐
   d. Flip angle ☐
   e. Matrix ☐

137. SNR is a factor that is measured.

   a. True ☐
   b. False ☐

138. CNR is a factor that is measured.

   a. True ☐
   b. False ☐

139. Factors that affect spatial resolution (resolution in "space" or detail) include all of the following EXCEPT:

   a. FOV ☐
   b. Slice thickness ☐
   c. Flip angle ☐
   d. Matrix ☐

140. Factors that affect SNR (signal to noise) include all of the following EXCEPT:

   a. TR ☐
   b. Field strength ☐
   c. FOV ☐
   d. Matrix ☐
   e. Hour of the day ☐

141. Center frequency is a factor that determines the:

   a. Frequency of RF used for excitation ☐
   b. Frequency of RF used for signal detection ☐
   c. a and b ☐
   d. Amplitude and/or duration of the RF pulse (to determine flip angle) ☐

142. Transmit gain is a factor that determines the:

> **a.** Frequency of RF used for excitation ☐
> **b.** Frequency of RF used for signal detection ☐
> **c.** a and b ☐
> **d.** Amplitude and/or duration of the RF pulse (to determine flip angle) ☐

143. Geometric accuracy is determined by the:

> **a.** RF system ☐
> **b.** Shim system ☐
> **c.** Gradient system ☐
> **d.** Main magnet system ☐

144. During MR imaging, all equipment should be inspected prior to use to be sure that components are in proper working order. Components include:

> **a.** RF coils and cables ☐
> **b.** RF coils and door seals ☐
> **c.** Cables and door seals ☐
> **d.** Quench system ☐
> **e.** All of the above ☐

145. Reducing the slice thickness by a factor of 2 will reduce the SNR (all other factors remaining constant) by a factor of:

> **a.** 2 ☐
> **b.** 1.41 ☐
> **c.** 2.5 ☐
> **d.** 1.5 ☐

146. The methods for shimming the main magnetic field are:

> **a.** Retroactive shimming ☐
> **b.** Active shimming ☐
> **c.** Passive shimming ☐
> **d.** b and c ☐
> **e.** a, b, and c ☐

147. The purpose of shimming a magnet is to:

> **a.** Make the B1 field as homogeneous as possible ☐
> **b.** Make the B0 field as homogeneous as possible ☐
> **c.** Make the scan times as short as possible ☐
> **d.** Correct for improperly tuned gradient coils ☐

Part D: Answers

1. c

2. a

3. b

4. d

5. a

6. b

7. c

Regarding questions 1–7: MR imagers are made up of a number of system components, each with its unique characteristics. Although we refer to the MR scanner as "the magnet", there are several types of magnetic field associated with each MR imager. These system components include the main magnet, the RF system, the gradient system, and the shim system (to name a few).

Within the MR system there is a "main magnetic field", also known as the "static" (or unchanging) field. This main magnet can be a permanent magnet (generally, heavy in weight, low field strength 0.3 T, open configuration, vertical field direction, always on), a resistive magnet [generally, lighter in weight, low field strength 0.3 T, open (or tubular) configuration, vertical or horizontal field direction, the only system that can be turned off when not in use, large energy (current) requirement], a superconducting magnet [generally, weight higher than resistive but lighter than permanent, high field strength 1.0 T, 1.5 T, 3.0 T, and higher, "tubular" configuration, horizontal field direction, always on, requires cryogens (liquid helium to make the magnet superconducting and liquid nitrogen to keep the helium cool) to maintain superconductivity], and/or a hybrid (generally, a combination of a resistive and permanent, or a combination of a permanent and superconducting).

The main magnet allows for the proton spins to align with the magnetic field. This process is known as magnetization. Another name for the main magnetic field is the primary magnetic field or B_0.

The RF system provides a means for excitation of the proton spins. Another name for the RF system is the secondary magnetic field or B_1. The RF system has a means for transmitting the RF signal (transmitter) and also receiving the signal (receiver). The RF transmitter "transmits" an oscillating radiofrequency signal. The oscillating magnetic field is known as a time-varying magnetic field (as the field "oscillates" or varies over time).

The gradient system provides a means for spatial encoding of the proton spins. Another name for the gradient system is the time-varying magnetic field (TVMF). The gradient system includes z (superior to inferior direction), y (anterior to posterior direction), and x (right to left direction). Gradient systems provide a means for selective excitation (slice selection), phase encoding, and frequency encoding (readout).

Each task (slice selection, phase encoding, or frequency encoding) can per formed with each gradient (*x*, *y*, or *z*). For example, if an axial slice is to be performed, the *z* gradient is used for slice selection and the remaining gradients (*x* and *y*) are used for phase encoding and frequency encoding. The phase-encoding direction typically defaults along the smaller matrix (to reduce scan time) and the smaller anatomy (to reduce phase ghosting artifact). For example, (regarding anatomy) an axial head would be phase encoded right to left; however, an axial abdomen would be phase encoded anterior to posterior. Direction of phase ending for anatomy is to be sure that any phase ghosting artifacts will occur along lesser anatomic structures. For example, (regarding matrix) if an image is performed with a matrix of 256×128 or 128×256, phase encoding will be along the 128 direction (regardless of the configuration 128×256 or 256×128).

8. a

9. c
Nitrogen is used in some magnet designs to insulate the helium cryostat. This reduces the amount of helium that boils off.

10. b

11. c

12. b
Regarding Questions 10 to 12: Faraday's law of induction states that if a magnet (or a change in a magnetic field/delta B, DB or ΔB) moves across a conductor (a wire, the RF receiver coil, or the patient), a voltage (a change in voltage/deltaV, DV or ΔV) will be created within the conductor. The stronger the magnet (ΔB), the greater the voltage. [The shorter the time, the stronger the change in voltage (ΔV).] Faraday's law of induction is related to the method by which signal is induced within the RF receiver coil. Induced voltage is dependent on the strength of the magnetic field and the rate at which it passes through the wire. Therefore, the stronger the magnetic field moving through the wire, the stronger the current produced in the wire

13. b

14. a

15. c

16. c

17. b

18. d
Also, increasing the current in the wires and/or reducing the space between the turns of wire increases the magnetic field strength.

19. b

20. a

This is because the secondary magnetic field (B_1) created by the RF coil must be perpendicular to the orientation of B_0.

21. d

Since the slice thickness affects voxel volume, changing the slice thickness will change the spatial resolution.

22. c

The selection of slice thickness by the technologist is determined by the anatomy to be imaged. Slice thickness is determined by the gradient amplitude (high amplitude slice selection gradient creates thin slices) and the transmitter bandwidth (tBW).. The tBW is the range of frequencies that is transmitted during slice selection. The wider the range of frequencies, the thicker the slice thickness. Thin slices are acquired with a narrow tBW.

23. d

The receiver bandwidth (rBW) is the range of frequencies that is "sampled" during readout (when the echo is sampled). Default rBW is approximately 16 kHz (±8 kHz)., Wide rBW is approximately 64 kHz (±32 kHz) or greater. Narrow rBW is approximately 2 kHz (±1 kHz) or 4 kHz (±2 kHz). Decreasing the receiver bandwidth increases the SNR, but also increases the chemical shift artifact seen on higher field strength systems.

24. a

25. b

26. a

Gradient coils are used to spatially encode the data; RF coils are used to produce various image contrasts by their timing. For example, in SE imaging, the timing between successive 90° RF pulses is the TR. TR selections determine the amount of T1 information (weighting) for a given image. In SE imaging, the timing between 90° RF and 180° RF pulses determines the TE (half TE). For example, if the time from 90° to 180° is 10 ms, the resultant TE is 20 ms. TE selections determine the amount of T2 information (weighting) for a given image. These factors determine image contrast in MRI.

27. c

The B_1 field refers to the secondary oscillating magnetic field created by the RF coil.

28. a

29. d

To maintain homogeneity (evenness) of the main magnetic field, "shimming" is performed. Shimming can be performed by the service engineer by passive shimming (using metal plates, shim plates) strategically placed in and around the main magnet) and/or active shimming (using current applied within shim coils). Shimming can also be performed by the technologist by adding current to the gradient coils (known as gradient shimming).

30. b

31. d

32. c

33. e

34. a

35. b

36. c

37. d

Regarding questions 30–37: Gradients are used in MRI for spatial encoding. Gradients have several characteristics, including strength (amplitude), speed (rise time), combined strength and speed (slew rate) and % of time the gradient can work (duty cycle). Amplitude is measured in G/cm (gauss per centimeter) and milliTesla per meter (mT/m), whereby $10\,mT/m = 1\,G/cm$. Typical gradients slew rates are of the order of 40–120 mT. The steeper the gradient, the smaller the FOV and/or the thinner the slice thickness and/or the higher the matrix (translating into higher resolution). Gradient speed allows for fast scanning. Faster rise times allow for faster imaging.

38. e

39. d

40. c

41. a

42. b

Regarding questions 38–42: RF coils are used in to transmit and receive MR signal. Receiver coils have a number of configurations including linear coils (one wire configures into a loop – generally a flat coil), quadrature coil (configured with wires (or electronic components) that are perpendicular to one another), Helmholtz pair (linear coils that are coupled or paired with one single receiver), phase array, and/ or multichannel (coils that are coupled or paired with one multiple receiver). RF receiver coils provide signal information from the "diameter" of the coil across and the radius of the coil deep. For example, in a 5-inch round (linear) coil, signal is detected from 5 inches across and 2.5 inches deep. This yields a sensitivity profile that appears like half of a circle.

43. a

44. b

45. c

Regarding questions 43– 45: In order to achieve "resonance" during MR imaging, there must be a "match" between the frequency of precession (the rate at which the proton "wobbles" within the magnetic field) and the frequency with which it is transmitted. To calculate this frequency the Larmor equation is sued. The Larmor equation is $\omega_0 = B_0 \gamma_2$ whereby ω_0 is the frequency, B_0 is the magnetic field, strength and γ is the gyromagnetic ratio (the spin angular momentum and the magnetic moment for a given proton.

46. b

47. c

48. a

49. d

Regarding questions 47–49: When a patient is placed into the magnetic field, proton spins (within tissues of the body) align with and opposed to the direction of the magnetic field. After a few seconds, a condition occurs whereby there are more spins in line with the magnetic field than opposed to it. This condition is known as thermal equilibrium. During thermal equilibrium there are more spins in the low energy state (known as "spin up" or "parallel", in line with the direction of the magnetic field) than the high energy state (known as "spin down" or "antiparallel", opposed to the direction of the magnetic field).

50. b

51. b

Regarding questions 50 and 51–: Protons within the body are "moving charged particles" and therefore behave like microscopic magnets. These tiny magnets have magnetic fields known as the "magnetic moment" (μ). In order to gain signal from protons within tissues of the body, patients are placed into the magnetic field. At this time, proton spins ("magnetic moments") align with or opposed to the direction of the main magnetic field (B_0) (along the z axis).

During thermal equilibrium, there are more spins in line with the field than opposed to it. This "excess" of spins (known as the "spin excess") in the low energy state forms the "net magnetization". The net magnetization is represented by a vector and forms the "net magnetization vector" (NMV).

52. b

53. d

54. a

55. d

56. d

57. b

58. b

59. c

Regarding questions 52–59:– To gain information from the tissues that protons "live in", energy in the form of a RF pulse must be applied. This RF pulse must "match" the frequency of precession. This frequency is determined by the Larmor frequency. RF pulses are applied with the appropriate frequency (the Larmor frequency), amplitude (strength), and duration (length of time) to "flip" the magnetization. This RF pulse is known as the excitation pulse. During the application of the RF pulse, spins from the low energy state absorb energy and enter the high energy state. This is known as "excitation".

During excitation, several processes occur including:

- Low energy spins enter the high energy state
- Spins begin to precess "in phase"
- The net magnetization is transferred into the transverse (x/y) plane.

After the RF pulse is removed, spins begin to recover back to the low energy state. This process is known as "relaxation". During relaxation several processes occur including:

- High energy spins return to the low energy state:
  ○ T1 relaxation, T1 recovery, spin lattice, longitudinal recovery or relaxation
  ○ In one T1 time, 63% of the original magnetization recovers and 37% remains
- Spins begin to precess "out of phase" or lose phase coherence:
  ○ T2 relaxation, T2 decay, spin–spin, or transverse relaxation or decay
  ○ In one T2 time, 63% of the original magnetization decays and 37% remains
- The net magnetization recovers to a position along the z (longitudinal) axis.

While the net magnetization "spirals" back to equilibrium, signal voltage is "induced" in the receiver coil. This signal voltage is known as the free induction decay (FID).

60. a

61. b

62. c

63. b

64. a

65. d

66. d

Regarding questions 60–66: MR images are acquired for the evaluation of T1 relaxation times, T2 decay times, and the number of mobile hydrogen protons within the area of interest. These are known as "intrinsic" factors and cannot be changed. To enable images with strong T1, T2 or PD information, extrinsic factors

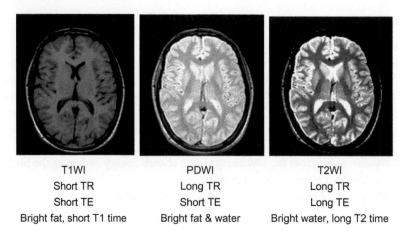

T1WI	PDWI	T2WI
Short TR	Long TR	Long TR
Short TE	Short TE	Long TE
Bright fat, short T1 time	Bright fat & water	Bright water, long T2 time

Figure D.1   Image contrast parameters.

can be manipulated by the system operator (technologist or radiographer). Extrinsic factors, which can be modified, can be used to manipulate image contrast based on T1, T2 or PD. These extrinsic factors include TR (for more or less T1 information) and TE (for more or less T2 information) (Figure D.1). Images acquired with short TR have more T1 information and vice versa. Images acquired with short TE have less T2 information and vice versa. TR and TE are selected as follows:

- Images with short TR (more T1 information) and short TE (less T2 information) yield images known as T1-weighted images (T1WI).
- Images with long TR (less T1 information) and long TE (more T2 information) yield images known as T2-weighted images (T2WI).
- Images with long TR (less T1 information) and short TE (less T2 information) yield images known as proton density-weighted images (PDWI) or hydrogen density- or spin density-weighted images.

Gradient echo (GrE) acquisitions are acquired with the selection of TR and TE (like spin echo sequences) and also the modification of flip angle. Flip angle goes with TR, which goes with T1. A short flip angle yields GrE images with less T1 information and vice versa. Since GrE sequences do not use a 180° RF pulse to create the echo (but rather use gradient pulses), the transverse magnetization "builds". This phenomenon is known as steady state. For this reason, the majority of GrE sequences are acquired as rapid T2* sequences. (FYI T2* = T2 + T2′ (whereby T2′ is associated with susceptibility, inhomogeneity, and chemical shift.) To remove the "steady-state" (T2*) effect, "spoiling" can be performed. This yields rapid T1 imaging for dynamic enhanced imaging or enhanced MRA sequences.

67. c

68. c

69. c

70. a

71. b

72. b

73. b

74. a

Regarding questions 67–74: Spatial encoding (or encoding MR signals "in space") is accomplished with the use of magnetic field gradients. Gradients are switched "on and off" during image acquisition. There are three "jobs" that must be performed to encode images along three dimensions: selective excitation (or slice selection), phase encoding, and frequency encoding (readout). There are three "sets" of gradients within the MR imager: the x, y, and z gradients. Gradients can be expressed as "physical" or "logical" gradients. "Physical" gradient is the term when the gradient is related to the physical body (and imaging planes acquired) and "logical" gradient when the gradient is illustrated on the timing diagram (Figure D.2).

When an axial image is acquired, the z gradient is used for slice selection (or selective excitation). In this case, the x and y gradients are used for phase and frequency encoding. The number of phase and frequency encoding steps is determined by the imaging matrix. For example, if a matrix of 256×256 is selected for imaging, 256 phase steps and 256 frequency steps will be acquired. Phase steps have a direct effect on scan time. For this reason, the number of phase-encoding steps is generally kept to a minimum. Therefore, for an image acquired with a matrix of 256×128 (or 128×256), the phase direction generally defaults to the smaller direction across the matrix. In this case, there will be 128 phase-encoding and 256 frequency-encoding steps.

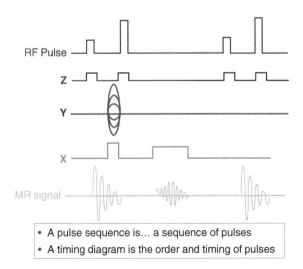

Figure D.2 Timing diagram.

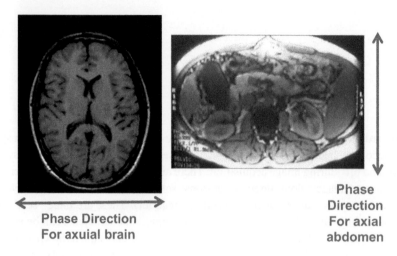

Phase Direction
For axuial brain

Phase
Direction
For axial
abdomen

Figure D.3   Phase direction.

In addition, motion artifact occurs along the phase direction (known as phase ghosting). Since motion artifact (or phase ghosting) occurs along the phase direction, phase encoding generally defaults along the short portion of the anatomy. For example, axial brain imaging defaults such that phase is right to left across the axial brain; but during axial abdomen imaging, phase is anterior to posterior across the axial abdomen (Figure D.3). For this reason, the direction of phase encoding is "generally" determined by the anatomy to be imaged and the desired scan time.

75. a

76. c

77. b
T2* is affected by inhomogeneities in the magnetic field as well as within the tissue.

78. d

79. d

80. c

81. c

82. b

83. c

84. d

85. c

86. a

87. d

88. c

The individual spins are precessing out of phase at equilibrium due to inhomogeneities in the main magnetic field and the effect of other spins.

89. d

90. b

The receiver coils are oriented 90° to the physical z axis.

91. b

The B_1 magnetic field is the field produced by the coil transmitting the RF pulse.

92. a

Although it is electromagnetic radiation, it is nonionizing.

93. c

Only some of the low energy spins enter the high energy state and the spins precess in phase. The net magnetization is therefore tipped into the transverse plane.

94. d

When the precessing net magnetization passes through the receiver coil, it induces a signal in the coil (Faraday's law of induction).

95. a

If 360° of phase change occurs in 1 second, then the frequency is one cycle per second (1 Hz).

96. b

97. b

Thinner slices are produced with higher amplitude gradients.

98. d

99. c

The gradient that is used to select the slice is the one that is oriented perpendicular to the desired slice plane.

100. b

101. c

To calculate the frequency required for excitation in MRI, the Larmor equation is used:

$$\omega_0 = B_0 \gamma$$

where B_0 is the static field, γ is the gyromagnetic ratio, and ω_0 is the frequency. The gyromagnetic ratio is 42.6 MHz/T for hydrogen. So, to calculate the frequency for 0.5 T, the equation is:

$$42.6 \text{ MHz/T} \times 0.5 \text{ T} = 21.3 \text{ MHZ}$$

102. d

The smaller the coil, the less the RF energy required for a given flip angle. The longer the duration of the pulse and the greater its amplitude, the greater the flip angle. Increasing the strength of the external field will increase the amount of power needed for a given flip angle.

103. a

The frequency-encoding gradient amplitude remains the same with each TR.

104. b

The frequency-encoding gradient is also known as the "readout" gradient.

105. c

106. d

107. d

108. d

When large FOV imaging is acquired, signals are "averaged", a phenomenon known as partial volume averaging. This results in a reduction in spatial resolution. When small FOV imaging is acquired, signals outside the FOV are "wrapped" around and onto the FOV in the wrong position on the image. This phenomenon is known as aliasing, wrap around, or fold over.

109. b

110. a

The undersampled tissue is "aliased" or "wrapped around" to the opposite side of the reconstructed FOV.

111. d

Some systems have an option that oversamples the FOV in either the phase or frequency direction (or both). The tissues outside the desired FOV are discarded and only the prescribed FOV is displayed. If this option is not available, the alternative is simply to increase the prescribed FOV.

112. d

113. b

114. c

The frequency difference between fat and water is field strength dependent. Lower field strength magnets do not produce images with very noticeable chemical shift artifact. The artifact is seen in the frequency direction as a dark and a bright line on opposite sides of structures with a fat–water interface, e.g. this is well pronounced on an axial view of the kidneys.

115. b

116. a

117. c

Because gradient echo sequences do not use an RF pulse to produce the echo, susceptibility effects are not corrected. Fast spin echo sequences use multiple 180° RF pulses and therefore correct for more susceptibility effects.

118. d

119. b

120. d

121. d

122. a

123. a

124. b

125. d

Regarding questions 121–125: Partial volume averaging (PVA) occurs as the voxel size increases. As FOV increases, voxel size increases and PVA increases. As slice thickness increases, voxel size increases and PVA increases. As matrix increases, voxel size decreases and PVA decreases. TR does not affect voxel size or PVA.

126. d

These are examples of methods available on most systems today for the reduction of motion artifacts.

127. a

128. a

129. b

130. b

Regarding questions 126–130: Motion artifact occurs due to periodic and/or aperiodic motion. Periodic motion occurs "periodically" (cardiac motion, pulsatile flow motion, and respiratory motion). Aperiodic motion is "random" motion (peristalsis and patient movement).

131. c

SNR is proportional to the slice thickness and square root of the number of signal averages ($\sqrt{4} = 2$).

132. b

133. a

134. b

135. c

Regarding questions 132–135: Signal-to-noise ratio (SNR) is the interrelationship between the wanted signal and the unwanted signal (or noise); this is a measured parameter. The relationship between the SNR of structure 1 (SNR1) and of structure 2 (an adjacent structure; (SNR2) is SNR1 − SNR2 = CNR. Contrast to noise (CNR) is a factor that is "perceived" or seen on MR images.

136. e

137. a

138. b

139. c

140. e

141. c

142. d

143. c

144. e

145. a

146. d

Active shimming uses coils that add to or subtract from the main magnetic field. Passive shimming uses pieces of metal strategically placed within the bore of the magnet.

147. b

B_0 is the main magnetic field.

MRI Calculations

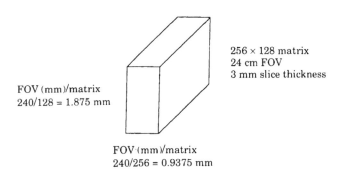

FOV (mm)/matrix
240/128 = 1.875 mm

256 × 128 matrix
24 cm FOV
3 mm slice thickness

FOV (mm)/matrix
240/256 = 0.9375 mm

$$1.875 \times 0.9375 \times 3 = 5.27 \text{ mm}^3$$

Isotropic voxel (3D acquisitions)

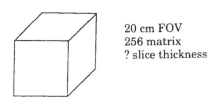

20 cm FOV
256 matrix
? slice thickness

200/256 = 0.781 mm
Slice thickness = 0.8 mm

Review Questions for MRI, Second Edition. Carolyn Kaut Roth and William H. Faulkner.
© 2013 Carolyn Kaut Roth and William S. Faulkner. Published 2013 by Blackwell Publishing Ltd.

Glossary of Terms and Abbreviations

Actual TE The time between the echo and the next RF pulse in steady-state free precession.

Aliasing artifact Produced when anatomy outside the field of view is mismapped inside the field of view.

Artifact A false feature in the image.

B$_0$ The main magnetic field measured in Tesla.

Bandwidth A general term referring to the range of frequencies contained in the signal passed by the processing system.

BUN Blood urea and nitrogen

Central lines Area of k-space filled with the shallowest phase-encoding slopes.

Chemical misregistration/shift Artifacts along the phase/frequency axes caused by the phase/frequency difference between fat and water.

Co-current flow The flow of nuclei in the same direction as slice excitation.

Contrast agent A substance administered to patients that alters selectively the image intensities of particular anatomic or functional regions, typically by altering the relaxation times.

Counter current flow Flow of nuclei in the opposite direction to slice excitation.

CNR Contrast-to-noise ratio: the difference in the signal-to-noise ratio between two points.

CNS Central nervous system.

Cross-excitation Energy given to nuclei in adjacent slices by the RF pulse – it is one cause of artifacts.

Review Questions for MRI, Second Edition. Carolyn Kaut Roth and William H. Faulkner.
© 2013 Carolyn Kaut Roth and William S. Faulkner. Published 2013 by Blackwell Publishing Ltd.

Cross-talk   Energy given to nuclei in adjacent slices due to spin lattice relaxation – it is one cause of artifacts that cannot be eliminated because it is the result of natural energy dissipated by nuclei.

CSF   Cerebrospinal fluid: monitored dynamically by ciné in patients with hydrocephalus.

CT   Computed tomography: the X-ray technique producing detailed cross-sections of tissue structures.

Decay   Loss of transverse magnetization.

ECG   Electrocardiogram: used to detect electrical activity of the heart; can be used to trigger the pulse sequence.

Echo train   Series of 180° pulses and echoes in a fast spin echo pulse sequence.

Effective TE   The time between the echo and the RF pulse that initiated it in steady-state free precession.

Entry slice phenomenon   Contrast difference of flowing nuclei relative to stationary nuclei because they are fresh.

ETL   Echo train length: the number of echoes produced and the number of lines of k-space filled, corresponding to the number of 180° rephasing pulses performed per TR.

Even echo rephasing   The use of evenly spaced echoes to reduce artifact.

FFT   Fast Fourier transformation: a mathematical process that converts the frequency/time domain to frequency/amplitude.

FID   Free induction decay: loss of signal due to relaxation.

Flip angle   The angle through which the net magnetization vector is rotated relative to B_0.

Flow phenomena   Artifacts produced by flowing nuclei.

FOV   Field of view: area of anatomy covered in an image.

Frequency encoding   A method of locating a signal according to its frequency.

Fringe field   A stray magnetic field located outside the bore of the magnet.

Gauss (G)   A unit of measure of magnetic flux density. The preferred SI unit is the Tesla (T).

Ghosting   An artifact in the phase axis produced by movement of the patient.

Gibbs artifact   An artifact commonly seen in the cervical cord as a result of truncation.

Gradient echo   The echo produced as a result of gradient rephasing.

Gradient echo pulse sequence   A sequence that uses a gradient to regenerate an echo.

Gradient spoiling   Technique that uses gradients to dephase magnetic moments.

Gyromagnetic ratio   The precessional frequency of an element at 1 T.

Inhomogeneities   Areas where the magnetic field strength is not the same as the main field strength – field unevenness.

Interleaving   A method of acquiring data from alternate slices and dividing the sequence into two acquisitions.

Intra-voxel dephasing   Phase difference between flow and stationary nuclei in a voxel.

K-space   An area where data are stored until the scan is over.

Longitudinal plane   The axis parallel to B_0.

Magnetic hemodynamic effect   The effect that causes elevation of the T wave of the ECG of the patient when placed in the magnetic field.

Magnetic isocenter   The center of the bore of the magnet in all planes.

MRA   MR angiography: method of visualizing vessels that contain flowing nuclei by producing a contrast between them and the stationary nuclei.

NMV   Net magnetization vector: the magnetic vector produced as a result of the alignment of excess hydrogen nuclei with B_0.

NSA   Number of signals averaged: the number of times an echo is encoded with the same slope of phase-encoding gradient.

Partial echo   Sampling only part of the echo and extrapolating the remainder in k-space.

Phase encoding   Locating a signal according to its phase.

Precession   The secondary spin of magnetic moments around B_0.

Proton density   Weighting image that demonstrates the differences in the proton densities of the tissues.

Recovery   Growth of longitudinal magnetization.

Residual transverse magnetization   Transverse magnetization left over from previous RF pulses in steady-state conditions.

Rise time   The time it takes a gradient to switch on, achieve the required gradient slope, and switch off again.

Saturation   Occurs when the net magnetization vector is flipped a full 180°.

Shimming   Process whereby the evenness of the magnetic field is optimized.

SNR   Signal-to-noise ratio: the relative contributions to a detected signal of the true signal and the random superimposed signals (noise).

Spin echo   The echo produced as a result of a 180°-rephasing pulse.

Spin echo pulse sequence   A sequence that uses a 180°-rephasing pulse to generate an echo.

Spin lattice relaxation   Process by which energy is given up to the surrounding lattice.

Spin–spin relaxation   Process by which interactions between the magnetic fields of adjacent nuclei cause dephasing.

Steady-state free precession   Excitation produced by strings of RF pulses applied rapidly and repeatedly at intervals that are short in comparison to T1 and T2.

STIR   Short TI inversion recovery: pulse sequence that uses a TI corresponding to the time it takes fat to recover from full inversion to the transverse plane.

T1 recovery   The growth of magnetization as a result of spin lattice relaxation.

T2*   Dephasing caused by magnetic field inhomogeneities.

T2 decay   The loss of magnetization that occurs as a result of spin–spin relaxation.

TE   Time to echo: the time between the excitation pulse and the echo.

Tesla (T)   The preferred unit of magnetic flux density.

TOF   Time of flight: rate of flow in a given time – causes some flowing nuclei to receive one RF pulse only and therefore creates a signal void.

Transverse plane   The axis perpendicular to B_0.